More Animals
in my Life

Also by Grant Kendall
The Animals in My Life

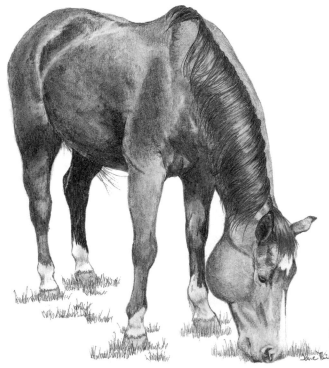

HOWELL BOOK HOUSE
New York

MORE ANIMALS IN MY LIFE

STORIES OF A COUNTRY VET

GRANT KENDALL

Drawings by Jane Thissen

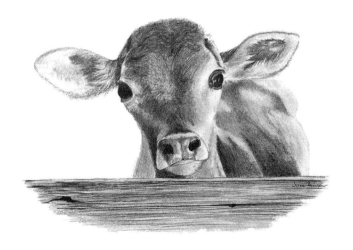

All the stories in this book are true, however, the names of the people and animals have been changed.

HOWELL BOOK HOUSE
A Simon & Schuster Macmillan Company
1633 Broadway
New York, NY 10019

MACMILLAN is a registered trademark of Macmillan, Inc.

Library of Congress Cataloging-in-Publication Data can be obtained from the Library of Congress

ISBN 0-87605-168-9

Manufactured in the United States of America
10 9 8 7 6 5 4 3 2 1

For Betsy

CONTENTS

$\mathcal{J}$NTRODUCTION

I HOPE ALL OF YOU WHO ARE READING THIS have read the previous book, *The Animals in My Life*, for two reasons: (1) There are a few references in this volume to incidents/animals/people in that earlier book, and (2) I need the money.

As in the first book, which actually is not necessarily prerequisite reading for this one, herein are stories of animals and the people who care for them. Some are funny, some are sad, and some are just stories, but all are true and taken from my quarter-century as a practicing veterinarian. Although most of these stories center on animals of various species, some are more people-oriented, but without the animals these people owned I would not have come in contact with them. People, after all, make up a good deal of a veterinarian's practice; never yet have I had an animal call me for treatment.

A few words and terms are peculiar to that profession and/or the horse business and rather than digress from a story to explain them, there is again a glossary included at the end.

I said in the earlier book that being a vet beats working for a living. It still does.

𝒫ART ONE

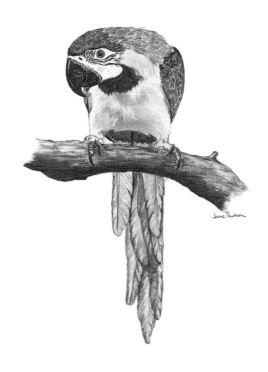

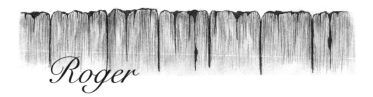

Roger

I'M ON RECORD AS SAYING I don't think wild animals should be kept as pets. Being taken from the wild as babies and forced to live in captivity is an adjustment many can't make, and their care is not easy. Many die, but worse, many do not domesticate, their owners grow to fear them, and they are "put to sleep," a ridiculous euphemism for murder. Fortunately, more people are realizing that owning wild animals is wrong, and it's not nearly as prevalent as it once was. And to help deter those who would still own them, laws to make it illegal are being passed.

That was kind of preachy. Sorry.

Some people also extend their dislike for the ownership of wild animals to birds. Sure, it's wrong (and illegal) to trap wild birds and sell them as pets, but the parakeets, finches, canaries, etc., that pet shops sell today have never seen the wild, no more so than the neighbor's Pekingese has ever seen ancient China or lived with its wolf ancestors.

The pet birds of today are domestic—bred, born, and raised in captivity for generations. Maybe it was wrong or immoral for the ancestors of these pet birds to have been captured, but maybe also it was wrong to catch and domesticate the ancestral horses, cats, dogs, cows, etc. That's a moral and ethical question I'll leave to deeper thinkers.

Back when we were first married and our living accommodations didn't allow for us to have a cat or a dog, we bought two parakeets. We named them Chicken and Dumplins, and they were good little pets, although hardly satisfactory substitutes for the dog and cat we really wanted.

They were extremely docile and agreeable. We'd let them out of their cage when we were home, and there was no fear of being unable to catch and recage them. Chicken, in fact, would often land on one of our heads or shoulders or hop on the couch beside us.

Dumplins was a little less people-oriented; her main out-of-cage activity was climbing the screen door and talking with the wild birds outside. She would chirp and a wild bird would chirp in reply. Sometimes the chirp patterns would vary, but there was little doubt that it was, indeed, a conversation.

Our daughter became a bird lover, and over the years she has had various parakeets and finches of her own. Whenever I see her walking around with one of her parakeets, I remember the first contact I ever had with a pet bird. His name was Roger, and he may well have been captured out of the Amazon basin or some other exotic spot, but neither I nor society thought much about it back then.

Roger was old. Fran said he was at least fifty, maybe sixty.

Fran was older. She was a 109. *109!* She had owned Roger at least half her life, she said.

Roger was a parrot, a big, green, red-faced parrot. I think he was probably a macaw of some type, but I have been told that macaws don't learn to speak easily, so I don't know. He sat on a perch in Fran's living room each day until her bedtime, when she would simply say, "Cage." He would repeat "Cage," then he would jump off the perch, waddle across the floor and through the door to her bedroom, hop onto a table, and go into his cage.

I know very little about parrots and parrot vocabulary, and Roger is the only parrot I've ever known, but he could speak as clearly as any person. He only said three things: "Cage," in response to Fran's bedtime command; "Cracker for Roger," presumably when he wanted one; and "Where's Jack."

Jack was—had been—Fran's husband, but he had been dead nearly forty years when we knew Fran. Whenever Roger would say, "Where's Jack" (it was never a question), Fran would answer, "He's gone now, Roger, but Jack will be back."

It was the early 1950s, and I was nine or ten years old. My grandmother, who was then in her late sixties, had more time than she could fill, so she joined a group of other retired people—six or seven of them—to help shut-ins. Somehow she had learned of Fran, who lived all alone except for Roger and her cats, on a run-down and neglected eighty-acre farm in the foothills a few miles out of town.

Fran was alert, bright-eyed, and mentally sharp. She could walk just fine, albeit slowly, but spent most of her time in a wheelchair because it was easier than walking. She couldn't drive, however, even though she had a car. It probably wouldn't run; it was a 1920-something Packard, and she hadn't driven it for more than twenty years.

For years, her friends, neighbors, and son would buy her groceries for her or take her places she needed to go, which weren't very many. She needed an occasional medical checkup, but in those days doctors still made house calls. But at 109, Fran was outliving all those who would help her. She was on her third doctor alone since Jack died.

As I said, Grandmother learned of Fran and began doing her shopping for her. I was usually recruited to help carry the bags, but I didn't mind because Fran was funny and Roger was neat. Grandma and Fran became friends—good friends. Sure, Fran was forty years older than Grandma, and if Grandma had been twenty or thirty it would have been an intimidating age difference, but at this point in their lives they were both old ladies. What's a few decades after you reach a certain point?

Her cats were an important part of Fran's life. She didn't know how many there were, but there had to be at least a hundred. Every one of them was feral. One, an old yellow tom, would come in the house but no one, not even Fran, could touch him. The other ninety-nine or so lived out on the farm—in old barns, in collapsing sheds, in a dilapidated silo, and in the old Packard.

But Fran loved them and fed them. Grandma said that half her grocery money was spent to feed those cats. Along the back of her house was a long screened porch, and that's where she would feed them. There were forty-four—I counted them—bowls, dishes, plates, pie pans, pots, etc., out there, and every evening between five and six she would totter out and fill each with cat food.

Grandma told me to do it once. "No!" Fran commanded. "They're my cats and I want to feed them."

Once the containers were full, she would open the porch's screen door and prop a chair against it to keep it open. Then she'd call, "Kitty-kitty-kitty! Here kitty-kitty-kitty!"

And cats would come. Like a lemming migration, cats—all sizes, shapes, and colors—appeared from the old buildings and streamed to the porch, where all the cat food was gone within minutes. Then they'd leave again, except the old tom, who would occasionally stay. It often earned him a few table scraps.

Television was just beginning then and Fran didn't have one. Grandma offered to buy her one, and my father said he'd put up an antenna, but she refused. She had a radio, and at that time there were still programs on such as *The Shadow, Mr. District Attorney, A Date with Judy,* and *Our Miss Brooks.* She spent her evenings listening to those.

And wasn't this the ideal entertainment medium? If a woman in a radio show was supposed to be beautiful, the listener could picture her in his mind as his or her idea of beauty. A handsome man was as handsome as the listener could imagine. If a bad guy was supposed to be evil, the listener could form his or her own idea of evil. Television has effectively killed imagination.

I visited Fran with Grandmother many times. I spent my time drawing or watching Roger as the two old women talked, but even though I was not con-tributing to the conversation, I would listen.

Fran spoke often of Jack. "He worked the farm every day, year-round, rain, shine, snow, or whatever. He'd come in for dinner, and if he was a little late, I'd say to Roger, 'Where's Jack?'" ("Dinner" was their midday meal.) "The same at supper. 'Where's Jack?' I'd say to Roger if he was a little late. It wasn't long before he'd say it, too. Dozens of times a day."

In these conversations, each time Fran said "Where's Jack?," Roger would look toward her and echo "Where's Jack." Occasionally, Fran would look over to the old bird, smile, and say, "Jack's gone, old Roger, but he'll be back someday." These were the only times her bright eyes would dim a little as a tear or two would form.

Fran told Grandma about her kids. "We had two children—beautiful children. I'd never have had any if I had known I'd outlive them." She'd smile a sad smile when she spoke of them.

"Johnny was such a good boy. Goodness, he's been gone over ten years now. He was only eighty-one when he passed away. He came to see me whenever he could but he lived almost a hundred miles away. He'd call two or three times a week. He was a wonderful son. He and Sharon were married sixty years but they never had any children. She passed within a month after he did."

Then she'd shake her head. "Rachel was beautiful, just beautiful, but Jack and me, we did something wrong. I don't know, she ran around. She married early—must've been seventeen or eighteen—but it didn't work. She was married five or six times, had five or six children, but I never heard from her or them. I used to write her and ask her to please bring her children to see me, but she never did. I'd get a Christmas card from her usually, no birthday card. Never a birthday card. Never a call.

"She was only sixty-something when she passed. Johnny came to tell me. He read it in the newspaper. I'm glad Jack wasn't still here then."

With every mention of Jack's name, Roger would squawk, "Where's Jack."

Fran must have told Grandmother the stories of Jack and their kids a dozen times. Most times when she spoke of her husband, even though there was a little tear, she would smile and tell Roger, "He'll be back someday."

"*Awrk.* Where's Jack."

Fran liked my drawings, or said she did. I drew and colored a picture of Roger looking at the old tom cat and gave it to her. She had Grandma bring some thumbtacks and put it up on her dining room wall "so I can see it when I eat."

She would let me give Roger a cracker when he would say, "Cracker for Roger." One evening when we stayed there late, she let me say, "Cage," but the old guy just looked at me and repeated, "Cage." Fran frowned at him. "Roger! Cage!" she ordered. "Cage," he said, and went straight to it.

But what he said most was "Where's Jack." People tell me parrots don't think—they just echo—but when Roger heard a noise on the porch—the wind blowing the screen door, the old tom scratching to get in—he would raise his head and say, "Where's Jack." It was never a question, always a statement. In a two-hour visit, he might say it ten times.

One afternoon after school, Grandma and I drove out to Fran's. It was after 6 when we got there, and the cats—most of them, anyhow—were milling around the door to the porch.

"Fran must be getting ready to feed them," Grandma said.

Grandmother never knocked, so we walked on in. Fran wasn't getting the cat food ready. She was just sitting in her wheelchair, smiling.

"Hi, Fran," I said.

She just sat there, not moving.

"Oh, no," Grandma said.

Fran was gone.

Roger had just been sitting there on his perch, cocking his head back and forth and looking at her.

"Want a cracker, Rog?" I asked, after I got over my dismay.

He perched quietly, just shuffling his feet slightly. He kept looking at Fran.

"Where's Jack?" I asked him.

He tilted his head at me. "Jack's back," he said.

Grandma notified the police, and they took care of Fran's body. She called the animal shelter and told them about the cats. We took Roger and gave him to a friend of my mother who wanted a parrot, but the old boy never adjusted to the new environment. They found him dead one morning several weeks later. All he had ever said in his new home was "Jack's back" a few times.

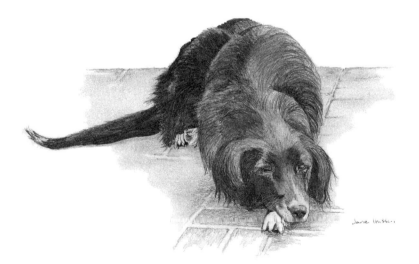

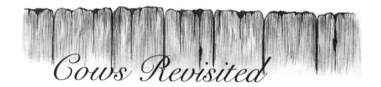

Cows Revisited

PERHAPS WHEN I WROTE *The Animals in My Life,* I left the impression that
I think all cows are bad. All *live* cows, at least. I heard from a reader (I hope he
bought the book and didn't just borrow it) who said I should not judge all cattle
by the few unfortunate experiences I had.

Well, I tried to let it be known in a story about our bovine friends (?) that
those incidents were just highlights from a myriad of cow-problem exposures, but
apparently there are those who came away believing those were my sole encoun-
ters with the fiendish creatures. Therefore, I wish to clarify my stance on cattle so
there will be no misunderstanding, now or in the future:

Cows are bad!

(When you picture a cow in your mind, what do you see? Two little
curved horns on the sides of the head. Cloven-hooved feet. A tail. Right? Now
picture Satan in your mind. Two little curved horns on the sides of the head.
Cloven-hooved feet. A tail. Coincidence? Hardly.)

Before we begin, to be fair (and Fair is my middle name), let me say that
all cow troubles are not necessarily the fault of the cow. Many of the problems are

directly related to management, but cows are what I ended up working on, so I blamed them. I know, it's sort of like shooting the messenger.

To be absolutely certain the world knows of the evils of cattle, I will now relate more tales of the distress and misery they have caused me, even though each of these brings forth painful memories. But I'm tough, so here goes.

Way back in undergraduate school—in the Beef Production course we were required to take to get a degree in animal science—we were taught how to turn a live cow into beef. Even though I don't like the former and do like the latter, I derive no pleasure from the conversion process, necessary though it may be.

This procedure involved using a chute and headgate and was performed indoors because the product had to be placed in a cooler. The room was large, perhaps forty feet by forty feet, and one side was partitioned into a holding pen large enough for perhaps a dozen animals, which were placed there through an outside door from a loading dock. From this pen led a short chute ending at the headgate. Overhead was a track from which the late animals would be suspended and transported from the headgate, because the trip into said headgate was one-way and the animal was rendered unable to walk out. Or do anything else. Supposedly.

Because of this, there were no cattle-confining structures beyond the headgate, just the remaining area of the large room and a normal-size entrance door for people to come and go.

The closure of the headgate around a cow's neck requires a certain level of coordination. Our particular class was not an especially coordinated one.

On that first afternoon we were to convert bovine into beef, our class gathered in the room with Dr. Strang. Most of our class, that is. There were only twelve members, so one absentee was easily noticed. Bill Minton wasn't among us.

We proceeded nonetheless. Two students climbed into the holding pen, chose an animal, and directed her—with difficulty—down the chute. This could have been a race cow; by the time she reached the headgate, she was approaching

MACH-1. The student manning the headgate was a nice but less than gifted soul named R T (I originally thought his name was Artie, but later learned it was just initials) who, under the best of conditions and with a stumbling, geriatric cow, would have had a tough time closing the gate properly and in time to catch the animal. With Lightning Lucy barreling down the chute, there was no contest. She burst through into the noncow-accommodating portion of the room and was tearing around the area in circles when Bill Minton, our missing classmate, showed up.

As he opened the door to come in, the cow saw her chance. She bolted for freedom, barely missing him.

"After her, boys!" commanded Dr. Strang.

The room was located in the Animal Science Building, which also housed offices and classrooms. There were two directions the cow could choose as she exited the room. To the right was a dead-end corridor. To the left was the open front door of the building and beyond that a campus filled with twenty thousand students, most of whom had never seen a cow outside of Kroger's meat department. And beyond that, the city. Guess which way she turned.

As she bolted through the front door, just missing a young woman who was entering the building, and out into the world, one student yelled, "We've got her now! She'll never go down the steps!"

She took the flight of fourteen steps in two easy bounds and headed across the campus, scattering students in her wake. Hot on her heels, but not gaining, was our class of a dozen animal science students.

One of my favorite spots on campus is a large lawn behind the Student Union Building, secluded from the road by two girls' dormitories. It is a favorite sunbathing area for the coeds who inhabit those dorms, and it is a favorite scenic diversion for the male students. We would make every attempt to pass through there on warm, sunny days to see the young ladies in their various skimpy sunbathing outfits.

This day was very warm and sunny, and our cow headed right through there. It was maybe a half mile from the Animal Science Building, but she had lost none of her speed. Our class, however, had, and our dozen were beginning to spread out considerably.

As she (and we) stormed across the sunbathing lawn, she scattered the variously underclad coeds, but none of us, her pursuers, were in a position to fully enjoy the sights. I was in the front line of pursuit and had no time to tarry as, naively, I believed we were gaining on her.

A large, thick hedge ran (notice I say "ran") from the edge of the Student Union Building to the edge of one of the dorms. Our cow was headed for it.

"Now we've got her!" wheezed and gasped Bill, who was a few yards ahead of me.

She didn't miss a beat. She tore right through the center of the hedge and out onto a main thoroughfare, and we tore through after her. Again, she was faced with two possible directions: left, which would eventually take her off campus, through a subdivision, out of town and into the countryside, where she could conceivably run free forever; and right, which would take her into the middle of a city of fifty thousand people. You know which way she chose, and we headed into town after her. She had to be tiring. I know I was, and several of my classmates were so far behind now they couldn't be seen.

After a few blocks, she decided there was too much automobile traffic in the street so she diverted to the sidewalk, where there was a lot more pedestrian traffic than I thought there should be at that time of day (why didn't these people have jobs?), but pedestrians didn't seem to bother her. They scattered.

"What are you doing?" yelled one.

I thought it was pretty obvious, so I didn't reply, but Bill, possibly raised with more manners than I was, panted back at him, "Chasing a cow!"

If there was further comment from the gentleman, we didn't hear it because we were still hot on the trail.

I clocked it later. It was 1.6 miles from the Student Union Building to Sam's News Stand, where we caught up with her. Sam's was an open-fronted structure that housed rack after rack of newspapers, magazines, and paperback books. It was about twelve feet wide and twenty feet deep, and for some reason our cow decided to enter it.

Bill was the first on the scene, and Larry Mallory, who later entered vet school with me, was right behind him. I was third and between the three of us we blocked the entrance to Sam's so the cow could not escape. She could have bowled us over, of course, but she, like us, was pooped. Over the next several minutes, the rest of our class wheezed in. Some of us were pretty out of shape.

As we stood there gasping and panting, R T asked, "What do we do now?" No one knew, so we continued to just stand there.

Fortunately, Dr. Strang knew what to do. He had not joined us in our pursuit. Instead, he had gotten a truck, a trailer, and the cattle herdsman, and a few minutes later they arrived. The herdsman walked right up to the cow, placed a rope halter over her head, and led her into the trailer.

"Okay, boys," Dr. Strang said as he got into the truck with the herdsman, "class is dismissed for today." And then he added, "Minton, be on time tomorrow. If you're late, you won't get in. The door will be locked."

By the way, Sam, of Sam's News Stand, was not happy. The school paid for the damage, quite a bit of which was done by the cow's digestive and urinary tracts emptying as we kept her confined in his shop.

Just a couple more examples of the difficulties cows can cause and we'll get on to real animals.

Dairy cows are afflicted with a condition called milk fever. At one time I could have given a long discourse on milk fever, but fortunately I haven't needed to know about it for so many years that I've forgotten most of what I knew. (Use it or lose it.) All I remember now is it involves calcium depletion in heavy milkers, and with low calcium, their muscles don't function properly and they go down and can't get back up.

Milk fever cases are easy to treat: Run a solution of calcium intravenously and the cow is better. It's easy because (1) the cow can't get up and run away, and (2) a cow's jugular vein is huge and easy to hit with a needle. To prevent her from flinging her head about, you put a rope halter on her head and tie it to a hind leg, then you pop a needle in the vein and run a half liter (I think) of the calcium solution into her system. In most cases, by the time the needle is removed from the vein the cow is struggling to rise. All health disorders should be resolved so easily.

The problem here lies with the time of day a cow needs treatment. For some unfathomable reason, the dairies in Richard's practice milked their cows at 4:00 A.M. (!) and 4:00 P.M. Maybe all dairies do this. Of course, if you plan to milk a group of cows at 4:00 A.M., you must first bring them to the barn, so you go to the field around 3:00 A.M. to get them in. And that's when the milk fever cases are discovered. And that's when the farm calls the vet. And that's when the cows have to be treated. A large Holstein dairy could have a dozen or more milk fevers a week.

I can't tell you how much fun it is to trudge out into a dark field with a flashlight at 3:00 A.M. to treat a down cow at Dairy A, then find a message on returning to the car that Dairy B, on the other end of the county (where else?), has one too. I never understood why they couldn't milk at 7:00 A.M. and 7:00 P.M.

One more, and this one was the one that really drove me to end my relationship with live cattle.

A very large Angus farm decided more beef could be produced if the Angus cows were bred to Simmental bulls. The resultant calves, it was reasoned, would have the beef quality of the Angus dams and the size of the Simmental sires. Angus are small, Simmentals are huge.

(My grandmother once told me a supposedly true story of a beautiful actress and a noted scholar. The actress asked the scholar to sire her child. "Think what a marvelous individual it will be!" she enthused. "It will have my beauty and your brains!" "But," countered the scholar in declining her offer, "what if it has *my* beauty and *your* brains?)

I don't know about the beef quality of the calves resulting from this cross, but at least the theory had been half right: They had the Simmental's size. They were huge, too huge, in fact, for the little Angus cows to give birth to them without help. A *lot* of help.

It's not unusual for a cow to need a little assistance in calving. A slightly too large calf or one that is malpositioned occasionally has to be pulled because the cow just can't push it out.

The results of these crosses, however, were not *slightly* too large to be pushed out. They were *way* too large. It was like trying to push a golf ball into a pop bottle. It just won't.

So we had to do C-sections. In themselves, C-sections in cattle aren't too bad. There is no critical time frame in which the calf must be brought into the world, unlike the case with foals; and cows, unlike mares, tolerate the surgery remarkably well.

This farm, however, had artificially inseminated its cows and timed the inseminations so the calves would arrive in March.

During this particular March, winter was hanging on. Days were only in the low forties and nights were dropping into the upper twenties. And nearly every day it rained. Well, not really rain—just a slow drizzle. You wouldn't get soaked unless you were out in it for an hour or so. The bone-shaking chill set in in about thirty minutes, though. And a C-section took thirty minutes to an hour.

In one seven-day period, ten of these poor little Angus cows attempted unsuccessfully to have calves as big as they were. I had to do C-sections on all ten. (One day alone there were *three*!) It took two weeks for my teeth to stop chattering.

By then I was on my way, family in tow, to a place where the only cows I would have to work on would be wrapped in cellophane. Someone should come up with a way to make beef some other way.

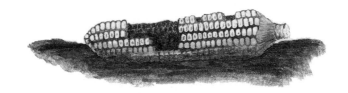

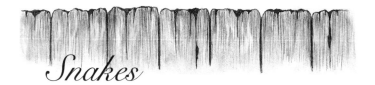

Snakes

I THINK I PROBABLY RATE SNAKES on a level near that of cows. No, maybe not. Cows have hurt me enough to where I have a little fear of them—or uneasiness, at least. Snakes have never done me any harm, so I'm not afraid of them. If I'm out for a walk and one scoots out of the grass or underbrush, I'm startled, but so am I if a rabbit or quail scoots out.

No, it's not fear, but I would just as soon a snake lead its own life and let me lead mine. This pretty much sums up my feelings about cows and slugs and bigots and many other lower life forms.

My earliest recollection of a snake was when I was about four years old, and I remember it not so much because of the snake but because of my parents. They had an absolute fit. I do remember that it was a pretty snake, though.

My brother, seven or eight years my senior (depending on the time of year), and I, out of boredom, would sometimes associate with each other. I preferred my friends and he preferred his, but there were times when we only had each other. Both of us liked animals, so we would occasionally go off into the woods to see what we could find. Our goal always was to catch something.

And we did, sometimes. Once Alan caught a squirrel, but it bit him and got away. Once I caught a rabbit, but it bit me and got away. Once we both caught a 'possum, but it "died" so we put it down. Then it got up, ran off, and climbed a tree. Basically, our bring-'em-back-alive safaris were marked by failure. And on those rare occasions when we actually did bring something home, we always turned it loose after we had showed it off to our parents.

One day, while searching on the back part of the property along the creek (or it may have been a stream or a brook or even a rill—I have never known the difference), Alan spotted a snake in the water.

"Let's catch him," he suggested.

"I don't wanna touch a snake," I protested.

"We'll put him in a bucket. Run to the barn and get one."

Today, I might tell *him* to run to the barn if he wanted a bucket, but at age four I was used to taking orders, so off I trotted. When I returned with the bucket, Alan had formulated a snake-catching plan.

"I'll hold the bucket sideways in the water. You take this stick and push him into it." He handed me a short stick. It was about half as long as the snake, which was every bit as long as I was tall.

Well, it sounded easy and it was. The snake bit my stick two or three times, but apparently finding it distasteful and unwilling to retreat, he turned and swam right into the bucket.

We had caught a snake! A real pretty sort of green-and-brown-striped snake! We ran home to show our prize.

We couldn't believe our parents' reaction. Our dad took the bucket from Alan and ran off with it. Later we learned he killed our snake.

Mother began crying and asking if we had been bitten. Were we sure? Let me see your hands!!!

When they calmed down, they told us it was a water moccasin. At the time it didn't mean a thing to us.

From that point until adulthood I had no further intentional snake contact. If I saw one, I said hi, but I didn't go out of my way to see any or speak to any. And they me.

I had one minimal snake contact in vet school. I'll tell you that story shortly, but first I want to tell you about an item that appeared in the newspaper a while back. Perhaps you saw it.

The headline in our paper read, "Pet python is killed to free pregnant woman, husband."

It seems the eight-months pregnant woman woke up at 10 A.M. to find "Calena, a (nine-foot-long) Burmese python, wrapped around her stomach and biting her buttocks." This is a direct quote from the newspaper, written, no doubt, by a science major. First, the stomach is an internal organ, and second, pythons do not "bite." The story went on to say that her husband, in attempting to free his wife, also became wrapped up by the snake.

This family, which also included two children ages four and five, resided in a one-room apartment. The husband was unemployed, yet they bought the snake for $150! I'm employed, and I can't afford a $150 snake. Also, the snake was not kept in a cage; she was allowed free slither of their one room.

Many questions were raised by the article: (1) Pythons only eat when hungry. Why weren't they feeding her? (2) How does anyone with a four- and five-year-old in the same county, much less the same room, sleep until 10 A.M.? (3) How did the woman get pregnant in a single room with a four- and five-year-old? We have nine rooms and doors that lock and our kids are older than those, but still the interruptions are sufficient to preclude pregnancy (or attempts at same). (4) Why didn't the snake go for the snack-size meal of one of the kids? A four-year-old is much easier to swallow than a grown woman.

Unfortunately, the outcome of this incident involved the demise of the python by decapitation at the hands of paramedics. The writer of the article expressed concern for the well-being of the people. What about the well-being of the snake? She was there by their choice, not hers, and she was evidently not cared for properly. I hope whatever animal welfare group they have in the city in which this occurred fully investigated and acted.

As an aside, I have a real problem with people having wild animals as pets. It's just not fair. When one acts according to its nature—i.e., eating when it's hungry or biting when it's scared—it ends up as Calena did: dead. Killed.

Now I'll tell you about the minimal snake contact I had while in vet school.

A classmate (Bob) and his wife (Shirley) owned a boa constrictor named Wally. This guy (Wally, not Bob) was five to six feet long and dearly loved. He had a cage but was usually allowed the wriggle of their mobile home.

Bob and I weren't really friends, but we studied together from time to time. On those occasions when we studied at his place, I got acquainted with Wally. As a snake, he was okay.

In our senior year, around Thanksgiving, Wally was gone when Bob and Shirley returned home from shopping one evening. They tore apart the mobile home looking for him. They canvassed the neighborhood. They placed notices in stores, called radio stations, put ads in newspapers. All to no avail. No one had seen Wally.

The couple brooded all winter. Christmas was no joyous occasion for them. "Wally was the best snake that ever lived," Bob wailed. I didn't know every snake that ever lived, nor, I feel, did Bob, but who was I to dispute that?

As winter progressed, I would often ask Bob if he had done a recent count of trailer park kids and pets. He was not amused.

One warm afternoon the following spring—some five months after Wally's disappearance—Bob and I and another student were at his place studying for an upcoming exam. Bob noticed some movement in a corner of the room. Investigating, he found Wally crawling out from a small space between the wall and the floor.

Bob was ecstatic! He called his wife at her work and she came home immediately. She was ecstatic! Wally's reaction was not recorded. He was, however, hungry. Bob ran out right away and ordered up a serving of white mice to go.

Apparently, when the weather in November had gotten too chilly for Wally, he had crawled into the insulation space between the internal and external floors of the mobile home to hibernate. A warm April day had roused him.

Graduation occurred two months later, and Bob and I went our separate ways to make our marks in the veterinary world (some days I think my mark is more of a smudge), and we did not keep in touch. I've seen no other newspaper stories similar to the tale of the ill-fated Calena, so I assume Bob, Shirley, and Wally lived happily ever after. Or else Wally swallowed them both and got away.

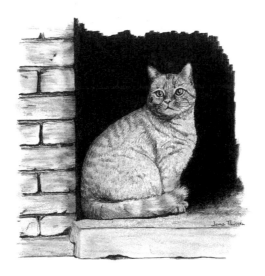

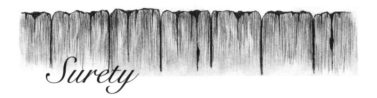

Surety

THERE ARE DISEASES that we can't cure and there are diseases that are incurable, and though they may sound the same, they aren't.

A disease we can't cure is one that gets out of hand, and death is the usual result. It can be an overwhelming infection or one that is ignored and goes untreated until it's too late. The latter we probably could have cured if treatment had been started when the first signs showed; the former may possibly have been cured, too, but the observer must be exceedingly sharp to catch the earliest signs.

A disease that is incurable is exactly that. There is nothing that can be done once the infectious agent—usually a virus—enters the host, be it a dog, cat, horse, cow, person, or whatever. Prevention is the key here; many of the diseases we can vaccinate against, but others we can only attempt to prevent exposure. Often, these diseases aren't fatal in themselves, but debilitate the host, sometimes to the point where death comes anyhow.

Equine infectious anemia (EIA) is one of these incurable diseases. Once a horse contracts EIA, if it doesn't die (which is unusual), it remains a carrier forever. A carrier, of course, is a source of infection for other horses.

Infection with EIA is acquired by entrance of the virus into the blood-stream. Obviously an infected horse (carrier) is not going to go around injecting other horses; the disease is spread by biting insects: Horsefly bites carrier, horsefly flits to another horse, horsefly bites other horse, other horse becomes infected.

(The largest outbreak of EIA, and the one that brought its potential danger to the fore, occurred at a New England racetrack in the late 1940s, but it spread there via a hypodermic needle that was used on many horses. A needle should be used only once and then discarded.)

Okay, infected horses don't die, so what's the problem? A big one: Red blood cells are destroyed by the virus (anemia), and infected horses become weak and depressed and lose condition. They become useless as working, racing, or pleasure horses. And if they live long enough, the anemia will do them in.

Control, then, is the key to EIA prevention. There is a blood test that can be done to identify horses that carry the virus. This is called a Coggins test, named after the person who first developed it. This test is required by law for interstate and international shipment of all equidae, and many states require it for movement within that state as well. Also, racetracks, horse shows, sales, etc., all require the test.

The fate of horses that test positive for EIA is unpleasant: They must be put to sleep or quarantined two hundred yards from other horses. Unfortunately, the latter is impractical or impossible in 99 percent of the cases.

Over the years I have taken hundreds, maybe thousands, of blood samples for Coggins tests and there have been positives. In my more than twenty years here in Kentucky I have had only one positive, but in the year and a half immediately after I got out of school I had a bunch. There are certain areas of the country where EIA is a problem, and the area I was in then was one of them.

The first positive was a month or so after I got out of school. It was a seven-year-old Thoroughbred gelding that was still racing but with a greatly reduced form in his last several starts. In his youth—at two and three—he had been a solid allowance horse, even placed in a stakes race, then he settled in as a hard-knocking $30,000 to $40,000 claimer, but had not won a race in four or five months, even though he'd been dropped all the way down to $10,000.

He was sound, and both the owner and trainer thought all he needed was a break from training, so he was sent to the owner's farm, which was a part of Richard's practice. He was to be there for six to eight weeks and then taken back to the track. The trainer sent the message that his Coggins test, required annually, would expire soon and asked that a new one be performed while he was at the farm.

The owner asked me to do it, and it came back positive. This explained his decreased racing performance. He had to be put down.

The last EIA positives I found there belonged to a young couple who owned eleven Quarter Horses—a stallion, six mares, and four yearlings. It was their third year in operation; two years before they had bought the stallion and mares and bred them, then foaled them out the next year. This was in early March; all six mares were in foal, and the couple was preparing to begin foaling. They were planning their future around the income the four yearlings would bring when they sold them later in the year.

One day I asked if they had current Coggins tests on their horses. No, only the ones they had when they bought them two years ago. Their yearlings had never been tested. I suggested they run the test on all their horses. They agreed.

All eleven came back positive. The couple was devastated. I don't know what the outcome was because I left for Kentucky while they were debating whether to attempt to quarantine all eleven. I imagine all their horses were euthanitized, though, because they weren't salable and never would be. I could have learned what happened, but I never tried because I didn't want to hear about eleven horses being destroyed.

Between those two instances there were a few other positives. No one was ever happy with a positive, of course, but they all understood. All except Bobbie.

A lot of the horse work in the practice was pleasure horses, and the boarding farms usually required at least annual and often semiannual Coggins tests for all their boarders. One such farm was owned and operated by an old lady named Mrs. Tutt, who probably forgot more about horses than most of us who care for their health will ever know. She required six-month Coggins testing, and anyone who didn't like it could take his or her horse elsewhere. Now.

Boarded on this farm was a Thoroughbred gelding named Surety. He was a very large, handsome chestnut of about ten or eleven years and was owned by an attractive but large (tall) young woman of maybe nineteen or twenty named Bobbie.

Surety's registered name was Social Surety, which made no sense to me; I think it may have been a play on words, but either it was too subtle for me to grasp or I was too dense. It didn't matter.

What did matter was Bobbie's love for him. No horse on the farm was better cared for, and this was a farm filled with little girls' and young women's pleasure horses. If reincarnation is real, that's what I want to come back as: a horse belonging to a teenage girl. Nothing is more loved or coddled or has a better life.

All the horses on Mrs. Tutt's farm were marvelously tended to—she insisted on it—but as I said, Surety's care was the best. Bobbie was out there with him more than any of the other owners were with their horses.

Bobbie had a severe socialization problem. She had been born without a left hand, whether she perceived herself as different because of this and because of her height (about six feet one inch) or because she was made to feel that way by her parents and schoolmates I don't know, but she chose to have her horse and Mrs. Tutt as her only friends. Surety was truly her life. She spent every moment she could find with him—riding him, grooming him, just talking to him.

One day when I was there for another young lady's horse, Bobbie was there, too, working on Surety. Both Richard and Mrs. Tutt had told me that Bobbie really didn't respond well to other people, so I always made it a point to go out of my way to be friendly, and she seemed to warm slightly. Later, Mrs. Tutt told me the reason she thought Bobbie accepted me better than most was because of my height; I was the only person Mrs. Tutt was aware of who had contact with Bobbie who was taller than she was (but only by an inch or so).

Regardless of the reason, this day, after I finished what I had gone there to do, Bobbie came out of Surety's stall.

"Dr. Kendall," she whispered very softly, her eyes looking down, "can I show you something?"

I stopped. "Sure," I said. "Is there something wrong with Surety?"

She said there wasn't and asked me to come to her car with her. There, she showed me a copy of Surety's race record.

"See," she said. "He was a good racehorse."

Well, he really wasn't. He had been unraced at two, possibly because of his size (very large two-year-olds often aren't ready to race at that age), but at three he had won two races and then another at five. He had been retired after that year with a record of thirty-some starts, three wins, and slightly more than $16,000 in earnings in the three years.

I told her I was impressed. I knew he had raced, but I had assumed it was unsuccessfully. Although his record was far from outstanding, it was better than I had imagined it would be.

Then she said, "I've got pictures."

I wasn't sure what she meant, but she reached back in her car and brought out three framed photos from his winning races. These may be purchased from the photographer at the track where the race was run, and they consist of a shot of the horse's crossing the finish line and another of him standing in the winner's circle with his trainer, owner, groom, etc. She hadn't owned Surety when he had raced—her father had bought Surety for her after he had been retired—but the pride could be seen in her face. I doubted whether she would have been any more proud if she *had* owned him then.

The fact that the pictures were framed I'm sure meant they were hung somewhere in her home. She had taken them down to bring to show me. I acted duly impressed and thanked her for showing them to me. She just smiled and went back into the barn to continue grooming Surety.

I got in my car to leave, but I realized I had left a used syringe and needle on a ledge in the stall of the horse I had been there to see. These aren't things to be left lying around, so I stepped back in the barn to retrieve them. Bobbie and Surety were in their stall three stalls down the aisle. I heard her talking to him, in a voice much louder and more assured than I ever heard her use in speaking to people.

I guess she didn't know I had come back in the barn, because she was saying, "He was really impressed by your pictures. Now he *knows* you were a great racehorse." I picked up what I had left and walked back out of the barn quietly; she was still talking to him.

The semiannual Coggins tests had been run by Richard a month before I went to work for him, so about five months after I got there I drew the blood from the twenty or so horses on the farm. All were negative.

In May, several weeks after Bobbie had shown me the photos, Mrs. Tutt called and said it was time for Coggins tests again. Surety had been there on the farm for three or four years and had been negative, of course, twice a year for that entire period, but this time he came back positive. The first I knew of it was when I received a phone call from a person at first so hysterical that I couldn't understand who it was or what was being said. After several minutes, though, the story unfolded.

It was Bobbie. The state veterinarian had called her and told her that Surety's Coggins test was positive, that he would have to be put down or quarantined two hundred yards from any other horses. He also told her he would be out the next day to take another blood sample to recheck.

Early in the call she accused me of switching samples, of mislabeling tubes, of contaminating Surety's sample with some other horse's blood. Then she stabilized a little and asked if there were ever false positives. Could there be a laboratory error? Would the lab see Surety's name on the retest and not even bother to run it, just mark it positive? Were there other labs?

I agreed to submit a new sample to another lab. I didn't know what else to do. I went there immediately to draw the sample, and I mailed it right away, before the state vet even came to draw his sample for the retest.

Well, of course, my second sample and the state vet's were both positive. Mrs. Tutt's farm was only twenty-some acres and there was no way Surety could be kept two hundred yards away from the rest of the animals. Bobbie called or visited every farm—literally—in a several-county area, and no one had, or would create, a quarantine facility. Anyhow, no one would take a Coggins-positive horse.

I have questioned my decision to become a veterinarian maybe twice over the years, and this was the first time. Surety was put down, but I couldn't do it. It had to be done by a vet made of sterner stuff.

Neither I nor Mrs. Tutt ever saw or heard from Bobbie again.

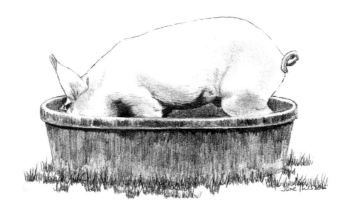

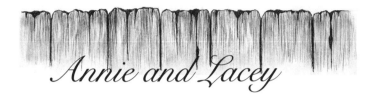

Annie and Lacey

I KNOW. THAT TITLE up there sounds like an old TV detective show, like maybe the little orphan girl grew up to be a cop. But it's not. It's about cats.

Actually, Annie got her name, sort of, from that little orphan girl. The first dog to bless our marriage was a small, black-and-tan, medium-coated mutt puppy whose mother had died when he was about two weeks old. For want of a better name, we called him "Orphan," but that very quickly became shortened to "Orf." And frequently, because he was very small when we got him, we referred to him as "Little Orf."

When Orf was about three months old, a friend had a litter of barn-cat kittens, a phenomenon we were to later experience to the fullest with Cat, but that story has been told. My friend's barn cat had only two kittens: a solid black male and a very light-grey-with-white-feet-and-belly female. I liked the color of the female, so I brought her home when she was barely six weeks old to surprise my wife.

She was delighted! (My wife, that is; the kitten just sat there digging her claws into my arm.)

"What shall we call her?" my wife asked.

"That's up to you. She's your kitten," I told her.

The whole time this discussion was going on, Orf was extremely interested. To our knowledge, he had never seen a cat, so I held the kitten down to him so he could sniff her, but I was prepared to protect her if needed.

It wasn't. Orf sniffed her for a moment, then began licking her. The kitten, initially digging her claws in even deeper, relaxed.

My wife said something like, "Little Orf likes her!" Then she said, "Annie! We'll call her Annie!"

Being slow at times, I asked, "Why?"

"Because we'll have Little Orf 'n' Annie!"

So she became Annie. She grew into a beautiful cat, one of the prettiest I've ever seen.

For a long time, we thought she was mute. We never heard her purr or meow. We could tell by her attitude and position of her mouth that she was meowing, but no sound ever came. She preferred me—cats have always taken to me—and one time when she was sleeping in my lap I happened to rub her throat. Although she was totally silent, I could feel the vibration there. She *was* purring.

Our worries about her inability to make noise were allayed one day when she was about six months old. This may actually have happened several times before, but it was the first we had seen. She was out in the yard when a neighbor's cat happened to stray onto our property. Annie didn't fight, but she growled and hissed and howled frightfully. Several other times we witnessed her in proximity (within a hundred feet) of another cat, and her reaction was always the same. She just didn't like other cats.

Early on she learned to use her sandbox and apparently came to feel that that was the only appropriate place to eliminate. When she was outside and the need came upon her, she would come to the door and howl until we let her in. If we were slow about acting, she would climb the screen door and shake it and howl. Once inside, she would zoom to her litter box, do what she had to do, and then request to go back out in the same manner in which she had requested entrance. No, she wasn't mute.

Annie wasn't spayed—there was no reason, I just kept putting it off (a responsible pet owner wouldn't)—but she never had kittens. I attributed it to her intense reaction whenever another cat was even slightly nearby; pregnancy requires a closeness she just wouldn't allow.

She remained an only cat for about three years. Even if we had wanted a second cat, we were sure it wouldn't work out. Cats react strangely, even aggressively, to other, strange cats, but Annie was the worst I'd ever seen.

One day a young woman we didn't know came to our door carrying a longhaired black cat. "Is she yours?" she asked. "We found her at our front door and we've asked everyone for miles. No one claims her."

We told her we'd never seen the cat before.

"She's very sweet," the young woman went on. "I'd love to keep her, but my husband is allergic to cats. I guess I'll take her to the animal shelter."

I hate it when anything is taken to the animal shelter, and I couldn't see this perfectly good and attractive cat going there.

"We'll keep her," I said, and we had another cat.

I took her from the young woman. She began purring immediately (the cat; the young woman left). About this time, Annie appeared from the back of the house.

"Look out," my wife said, "there may be a fight."

The black cat in my arms just lay there limply, purring. Annie stopped and looked straight at us.

"Put her out for now," I told my wife, but Annie jumped across the room and sat at my feet, making her soundless "meow" face. There was no hissing or growling. The black cat may as well have been dead for all she moved.

My wife picked up Annie to put her out, but she (Annie) leaned over toward me and the new cat.

"Bring her closer." I said.

She did and the black cat lifted her head and looked at Annie. Annie just stared back.

We put both cats down. The black one just sat there while Annie sniffed her from one end to the other, then grabbed her head with both paws and started licking her.

And that was all there was to it. No growls, no snarls, no hisses. The two became almost inseparable; wherever Annie went, the newcomer was right there. When Annie wanted out, the other one wanted out. When Annie howled to get in, her black friend was right there with her. They slept curled up together in a ball.

The new cat was given the name Lacey because my wife said she was as black and as soft as black lace. Lacey had the personality of a turnip. She was sweet and gentle, but that was all she ever did: be sweet and gentle. And followed Annie around like a shadow.

Somehow, though, she was a bad influence on Annie. After all the years of no babies, about two months after Lacey's arrival I noticed Annie was getting fat. And there was some development of her mammary glands. She was pregnant. She had still acted her same old way (or so we thought) whenever she saw another cat (besides Lacey), so I don't know how it happened. Well, yes, I do know *how,* but I really couldn't picture a tom cat getting that close to her.

About a week later, I noticed Lacey was also broadening. She was pregnant, too.

Annie's pregnancy resulted because I had just put off spaying her—laziness, I guess—but Lacey's condition came about because I just plain didn't even think about spaying her. It never crossed my mind. That's pretty dumb, I know.

About ten days after I noticed Annie was pregnant (and two or three days after I saw Lacey was that way, too), we were peacefully sitting at home one Sunday afternoon when Annie began pacing. I thought maybe she wanted out, but before I could open the door she went to the bottom shelf of a bookcase and lay down. Lacey went with her. (There were only two books on the shelf.)

A few minutes later my wife said, "What's Annie doing?"

I looked over at her. She was giving birth to a kitten right there on the hard wooden shelf. She seemed unconcerned and Lacey seemed fascinated.

Within twenty minutes, she had delivered three kittens. As they were born, she licked them and chewed off the umbilical cord, and as she lay back for more uterine contractions, Lacey would take over the licking. Annie didn't mind.

When the birthing process was completed, Annie gathered her three babies to her belly, and Lacey lay right there with them. The two took turns licking and cleaning the kittens. Lacey, it appeared, would be a good mother herself, maybe within the week.

But it wasn't that long. My wife placed a bath towel under the cats so they would be more comfortable and she called me over.

"Take a look at Lacey," she said.

Lacey was starting to have a kitten. She eventually had four—prematurely. They were small and weak and just not ready to be born yet. Two died within minutes, one lasted about an hour, and the fourth lived until the next day. I fed it with an eyedropper, but its sucking and swallowing reflexes were almost nonexistent.

I don't know if the stimulation of Annie's delivery had initiated the same process in Lacey or if it was an abortion that was just timed peculiarly, but Lacey seemed to think that Annie's kittens were hers. Or at least, partly hers. She helped Annie nurse them. In fact, when Annie decided she wanted a break, Lacey would stay with the three kittens and they would nurse her. Rarely has any litter been fed so well.

We found good homes for the three by the time they were six or seven weeks old, and, stupidly true to form, I didn't think about spaying.

A few months later, it was obvious that Annie was pregnant again. I checked Lacey closely, but I didn't think she was. Thank goodness.

Barb kept a towel on the shelf this time, and Annie delivered there—four kittens—one evening while we were out. When we came home, the two adult cats were surrounding the four newborns, and all seemed very happy.

When I checked them a little while later, I found Lacey on the floor in front of the shelf, lying flat on her side with her abdomen pumping heavily. I couldn't find anything wrong with her, but then I looked at her rear end. With each straining motion of her abdomen, a small portion of vagina prolapsed through her vulva.

I called my small-animal vet friend. "It sounds like a dystocia," he said.

"She's not pregnant," I said.

"Are you certain?"

"Almost."

He came over. Yes, she was not pregnant, he said, but "she sure looks like she's trying to give birth."

He sedated her, but she wouldn't stop straining. She died the next morning. My friend did a postmortem exam on her and could find nothing abnormal. I assume she somehow was triggered into "labor" by Annie's delivery. After all, it had apparently happened before.

Annie searched for Lacey for weeks. Many times I saw her go to the living-room chair where they often slept together and sniff around it and even look behind it. They had spent a lot of time in the guest room, and Annie would go there, jump on the bed, look under it, and sniff at the closet door. She'd prowl around the basement at length.

She managed to raise her kittens by herself. Almost. One died, but the other three went to good homes. In retrospect, we should have kept one for her. She was spayed shortly after her last kitten left, and until her death years later she never made friends with another cat, even though we had several others while she was still with us.

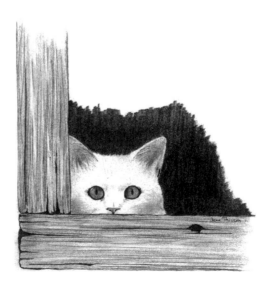

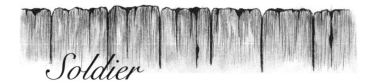

Soldier

As I was growing up I really liked animals, which in my immediate world consisted of dogs, cats, horses, the occasional goat, and various wild critters whose paths I would cross from time to time. Intentionally. I've probably said all this before.

There were animals I probably should have been afraid of, or at least had a little respect for what they could possibly do to me, but I wasn't and I didn't. I never thought about it. I liked them, why shouldn't they like me?

But when I was six or seven, I met an animal I *was* afraid of. Not at first, though; at first I really liked him, just as I really liked all the animals I came across.

He was a Doberman Pinscher named Graf, and he belonged to our next-door neighbor. Living on a small farm (farmlet?) as we did, that meant maybe an eighth of a mile away. Graf would come over to our place to play with Robin, our Cocker Spaniel, so I saw him a lot. He was three times Robin's size, and even though both were males, he was never aggressive toward him. He didn't chase the cats or bother the horses, and he was friendly to the people, so my family didn't mind his visits at all. I enjoyed them.

If he stayed too long—by his owners' standards, not ours'—a loud "Graf!" from his master or mistress was all that was needed to bring him home. He was a good dog.

One day—a very windy spring Saturday—my brother and I decided we'd go for a ride on his horse. We didn't do this often because he was a big kid and I was a little one, but I liked it. He would steer and I would sit behind him and hold on.

Usually, we would just ride around on our property, but sometimes Alan would take Captain down the road—on the shoulder. That's what we did on this particular day.

We rode past Graf's home and maybe a mile beyond, then turned around and headed back. The wind kept blowing things across the road, but nothing ever bothered Captain. He just plodded along.

When we were passing Graf's home on the way back, a big gust of wind blew my cap off and into Graf's yard. Alan stopped Captain, and I hopped off and ran after my cap, which had come to rest about twenty feet into the yard.

I assume when Graf saw me running toward his house he took it as a threat. He came at me and there was no mistaking his intent. He wasn't barking—he was snarling and his ears were flat back.

"RUN!" shouted Alan.

Perhaps if I had stood my ground and let him see who I was—after all, he knew me well—everything would have been all right. Or perhaps he would have eaten me. We'll never know because I did what Alan had ordered: I ran. Alan reached down and began to pull me up onto Captain when Graf caught me.

He had just bitten into my left ankle when we heard a loud, sharp "Graf!" and he let go. His mistress had seen what was happening.

Fortunately, Graf was marvelously well trained. Any time his master or mistress said his name, he responded immediately.

The lady came to see how I was. If I had been hurt as badly as I sounded—I was crying and screaming—I would have been at death's door, but all I had were a few little tooth holes in my ankle. They were bleeding, and when I saw the blood, I cried and screamed even louder.

Graf continued to come over and play with Robin, but when he was there I stayed out of the way. I was afraid of him, and it was years before I felt comfortable around a Doberman again.

In fact, I was in vet school before I made friends with another Doberman. Dick Bernard was a classmate, and we both had an interest in horses, so we gravitated to each other. We became good friends, and our wives became almost inseparable. Dick and I studied together a lot, and they'd come to our place or we'd go to theirs once or twice a week. (Dick's interest in horses faded for some reason. Today he has a huge consulting swine practice; people from all over the Southeast call him with their piggy problems.)

Dick and Marie had two dogs: a Chihuahua named Pablo and a Doberman named Rollie. For a Chihuahua, Pablo was a pretty good little dog, but it took quite a while for me to warm to Rollie.

I wasn't afraid of him or any of his breed anymore, but I didn't like Dobermans. Maybe it was mistrust, I don't know, but I do know it took time for me to accept Rollie.

But with time, I did. He was always glad to see me, and I came to realize he was very intelligent. Toward the latter days of vet school, I was very fond of the old boy. Several years after we were out of school we received a note from Dick and Marie that Rollie had died. I was sorry to hear it.

Still, I was not in love with Dobermans. Even knowing Rollie and seeing him at least a couple times a week for most of four years, I didn't care for the breed. When I was on clinic duty my last year of school and someone would bring in a Doberman, I would arrange for another student to take that case.

Then I graduated, moved, and began working for Richard in his vet practice. Richard owned a Doberman named Buford. Buford was enormous! He must have weighed 120 pounds, which was unfortunate because he thought he was a lap dog. He loved to crawl up in a person's lap, and he loved to receive affection and be loved on. He was an absolute sweetheart. And as with Graf and Rollie, he was very intelligent. And as with Rollie, I became very fond of him.

Next, we moved to Kentucky and I began my own practice. Eventually, I gained a client named Simon Landholder who owned a small breeding farm, a few horses in training, and two Dobermans, a male named Sentry and a female named Sonya.

Even though both dogs were mature—Simon said Sonya was three and Sentry was four—they acted like puppies: happy, frolicking, loving. But when Simon spoke, they listened and obeyed. Again, these were very intelligent dogs. I was coming to the conclusion that the Doberman breed is a pretty smart one.

We had finally put enough money aside to buy our farm (or I should say, make a down payment on it; the bank owned it). Shortly after we moved to it, Vichy, the old St. Bernard we had had since before I entered vet school, died. For a Saint she was old: eleven. Giant breed dogs really don't live long enough.

We were living pretty far out in the country and I was gone long hours. My wife said she'd feel safer if we had another big dog, so we talked about which breed we'd like. Even though we had loved Vichy dearly, we ruled out Saints for two reasons: (1) their coats require a lot of work; and (2) they're a wet-mouthed breed, and we had been slobbered on just about as much as we could stand.

We decided, therefore, on a shorthaired, dry-mouthed breed. She suggested a German Shepherd. No—too many problems brought about by indiscriminate breeding. Labrador Retriever? Maybe, but they're generally too good-natured to be much of a watchdog. Rottweiler? Gee, I don't know. Are they wet-mouthed or dry?

We discussed it for a few days and no decision was reached. My wife brought home a copy of *Dog World* and we looked through it. German Shorthaired Pointer? Rhodesian Ridgeback? We couldn't decide.

A few days later, I was at Simon's farm. It was October, and with the breeding season over I wasn't going there (or anywhere) very often. It had been three to four weeks since I'd last been there.

Sentry and Sonya were happy to see me, as usual. Why hadn't we considered Dobermans? I asked myself.

Sonya wasn't quite as exuberant as she usually was. I looked at her. She had gotten fat since I had last seen her. I said as much to Simon.

"Well, she should look fat. She's due to whelp in about ten days."

"She's gonna have puppies?"

"That's right."

"You gonna sell 'em?"

"Sure."

"Can I buy one?"

Of course. He was going to sell them for $300 apiece, but I could have one for $200. I told him I'd check it out with my family.

"You told me the only animal you've ever been afraid of was a Doberman," my wife said when I asked her if she'd like one. (I had never told her about cows.)

"I've changed my mind."

"I like Dobermans. I would have suggested one days ago if I had known," she said. "Tell me these things."

Ten days later Sonya gave birth to nine little Dobies. We took the kids to see the puppies when they were three days old. Our daughter wanted to take one then.

We saw them again at about two weeks and then at three or so. Each kid had a different choice. At five weeks, my wife liked one male in particular. At seven weeks, she liked him even more and so did I. He wasn't the largest of the puppies, but he was certainly the best-looking to our untrained eyes, and the most outgoing. Simon told us he was the pick of the litter, but I suspect he would have said that about whichever one we liked. We're easy, so we said he was the one we wanted. A week later we took him home.

It was December 20 so he became a Christmas present to ourselves. Our son wanted to name him Killer, our daughter liked Sweetie, and I wanted to call him Rebel. Barb really liked Soldier, and because she was the one who chose him in the first place, he became Soldier.

All my life I had been taught that animals need a brain to function. I no longer believe that. Soldier functioned—not obediently or reasonably, but he functioned. And he had no brain. He couldn't have.

He didn't housebreak. He ate furniture. He even ate the linoleum floor when we closed him in the kitchen one day. He'd wander off our property and not come home. We'd call him and he wouldn't respond. He chewed our shoes.

He chased the cats, but he wasn't quick enough or coordinated enough to catch them. He chased birds. He chased cars. He didn't want to be held or even petted. He would avoid the kids at all costs.

Nothing worked with him. We tried three or four training methods and they all failed.

Then one day he doomed himself. He began chasing the horses. He had to go.

I thought there would be protests, but he had chewed up enough of the kids' toys to where they were all for it. The kitchen floor had been the determining factor for Barb.

I wasn't sure what to do with him. He was eight months old, and an eight-month-old puppy is hard to find a home for.

Wilmer Brown brought us a load of straw one day. Wilmer lived across the county and supplied most of our hay and bedding. He was a good ol' country boy, with the stress on the "good."

That day he had a medium-size young mongrel with him. She was black and white with a medium-length coat. Wilmer had never brought a dog with him before, so I asked, "What's with the dog?"

"Found her on the way here," he said. "She was at the four-way stop in Centerville and every car that stopped she'd run up to. I figured somebody'd just put her out there and left her. I was afraid she'd get run over if she stayed there, so I let her in with me."

The dog jumped down out of the truck's cab, ran up to Cat, our barn cat, and began licking her. My son came to the barn and she ran over to him. She rolled over and let her stomach be rubbed.

"Don't really want her," Wilmer went on. "I'd really rather have a dog like that one you got there." He pointed to Soldier running frantically after some low-flying starlings. "He's beautiful, but I can't afford a fancy dog like that."

We traded on the spot. We named the mongrel Squirrel, and she grew to be medium-size and medium-coated, but at least she was dry-mouthed. She was intelligent and alert and protective and loving and didn't chase cats, birds, horses, or cars. She didn't eat furniture, toys, shoes, or floors. She was a great dog.

One day when Wilmer delivered a load of hay, he saw Squirrel and said, "You know, that Doberman I got from you is the dumbest dang animal I ever saw."

At least I'm not afraid of them anymore.

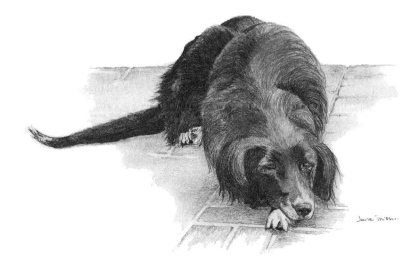

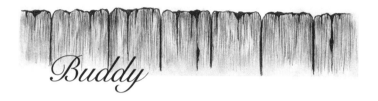

Buddy

"CAPRICIOUS" IS ONE OF OUR most distinctive and descriptive words. We have no words such as "equicious," "bovicious," "canicious," etc., because, I guess, horses, cows, dogs, etc., don't do anything as remarkable or whimsical or unpredictable as goats.

We had the occasional goat when I was small, but we never had one for long. I never knew why then, but I think I may now: Confining a goat is a challenge.

I remember liking the goats, but I also remember that they played pretty rough. I don't remember anyone else being abused by them, but they would always bat me about pretty mercilessly. Part of the reason, I'm sure, was that I was the smallest person they came in contact (a very fitting word) with and the least able to fight back. Still, even though I knew I would be butted and run over, I enjoyed playing with them.

After those early goats, my life was goatless for many years, until well into vet school. There we had to learn ruminant anatomy, so the misguided few who chose to enter cattle practice would know about such things. Cattle, however, are big, expensive, space-occupying, difficult to clean up after, and need lots of groceries.

A ruminant is pretty much a ruminant, however. I guess we could probably have used a yak or a zebu if either were plentiful, cheap, and easy to maintain, but they aren't. Goats are, though, so goats are what vet students use to learn ruminant anatomy.

And we learned, more or less. I'm fairly sure I learned less. But the goats were fun.

The goat assigned to our group was a nanny that happened to be pregnant. In the process of our learning, she aborted twin kids, and she had no milk. Another group also had a pregnant nanny that delivered a kid that same day and she had milk, so we borrowed some colostrum from her for our twins, which were small and weak.

There are very few things in this world as cute as a baby goat. And as sweet. They outgrow the sweetness very soon, but for the first few days, they are very loving little things.

And these twins were. As I said, they were small and weak and needed a lot of attention and TLC, so Shirley Gordon, one of our group, and I each adopted one. We took them home at night so we could bottle feed them often and then brought them back to school the next day because there was no one to care for them at home then.

They did well. We had no way of knowing when the nanny had been bred, so we didn't know how premature they were, but it couldn't have been more than a week or so. By the time they were two weeks old mine was ready to make it on his own. He was placed in a small pen in the food animal clinic and fed from a bucket. Shirley's was slower to come around, but by three weeks he, too, was on his own and placed in the pen with his brother.

That was the end of my goat experience in school, but when I went to work for Richard, one of the first things he told me about was his goat clients.

"I hate to tell you this," he began. "If I'd have said anything about it when I hired you, you probably wouldn't have accepted the job."

Golly, I thought, does he want me to treat an alligator farm or something?

"Grant," he continued solemnly, "there are two goat dairies in the county and I'm the vet for them. I don't like goats, so I'm going to have you do their work." He paused, smiled an apologetic grin, and said, "Sorry." He looked as if he was telling me my best friend was terminally ill.

"Great," I said. "I like goats."

Goats have far fewer problems than do cattle, and tending to their health needs was easy. The only bad thing about them was the odor of the mature billy goats. They really stink, and after you handle them the smell really clings to you. One of the goat dairy owners was very active in 4-H and had me come to a couple of meetings and speak to the members on goat health problems. I enjoyed it. When I left Richard's practice, the goat folks were sad to see me go.

I thought that with my departure any goat contact was behind me, but that was not the case. When I began practicing in Kentucky at the training center, I found there were goats everywhere.

Horses in training spend most of their time in stalls. It may be as much as twenty-three hours some days for a healthy, sound horse. An injured horse may actually be confined to its stall for weeks while the injury is healing. They get lonely and bored and they respond to that boredom in different ways. Some constantly walk circles in the stall, some kick the walls, some weave (constantly shifting weight from one front foot to the other while moving the head back and forth with the weight shifts), some rear up to look over the wall to see the horse in the next stall.

One of the tried-and-true methods of stopping all this (nothing is foolproof, however) is to give the lonely horse a companion. Another horse would be ideal, of course, but that's impractical, and besides, two horses will hardly fit in a twelve-by-twelve box stall. Therefore, other species are used. Over the years I've seen dozens of racehorses with smaller companions. One horse had a rooster, another a hen. One had a duck, one had a sheep, one had—believe it or not—a descented skunk. I read once of one that had a donkey for a companion. A few had cats, but cats seem to be the least satisfactory because they roam too much.

I remember two that had dogs. Late one evening I was called to the training center to treat a colic, and I passed the stall of one of these that had a dog companion. They were both lying down asleep, with the little dog curled up under his horse's throat, his head resting on the horse's.

The most common companions by far, though, are goats. I'm not sure why this is; perhaps it's because they're cheap and easy to care for. I imagine in the time I did track work I saw forty to fifty horses with goat companions.

The horses come to depend on their goats, and vice versa. The training center is just that—a place to train horses—and if a horse was to race, it had to be vanned to the track where the race was being run. Keeneland Race Course is in Lexington, so to run there a horse has to van only twenty minutes or so, but some are vanned 150 miles to race and then vanned back after the race. I have known a dozen horses that *had* to have their goats vanned with them.

Most of the goat companions don't like it when their horses leave. They call and bleat and run in circles until their friends return. Once a goat that dearly loved her horse got out of the stall somehow after her horse had left for a race. She ran throughout the entire training center crying for him. No one could catch her until six hours later, when her horse returned. Then she ran right to him and followed him back to their stall. On future race days, she rode along with him.

There was one goat that was extremely protective of her horse. Her name was Molly; she wore a dog collar and had to be tied or held whenever her filly left the stall for any reason. Also, she had a reputation for attacking anyone she thought was doing a disservice to the filly, whose name was Flitter Fry. (I don't know what it means, either; it may well have been a typo on the name registration form.)

I was the trainer's vet, and whenever I or the farrier needed to work on Flitter Fry (say it five times fast), he would either tie up Molly or have one of his grooms hold her. Usually he snapped a rope, which was attached to one of the rings that supported the feed tub, to the goat's collar. She hopped about and bleated and even turned somersaults trying to get free to protect her filly.

One day Flitter Fry came back from her morning workout with a slight limp. Anthony, her trainer, asked me to look at her. With a groom holding Molly,

Anthony led the filly out and I saw she was slightly off in her right foreleg. I told him to put her back in the stall and I'd examine her.

The first thing he did when he reentered the stall was to attach the rope to Molly's collar.

"Okay, Doc, now you can come in."

I bent down to feel the filly's ankle and foot for heat. As soon as I touched Flitter Fry, Molly began jumping and bleating and straining against the rope. I picked up the foot, and the next thing I knew I felt excruciating pain and, just like in the comics, saw stars—briefly. Then everything went black.

When I saw light again, I was sitting back against a bale of hay in the aisle outside the stall.

"Are you okay?" Anthony asked.

It took a second, but I finally replied. "What the heck happened?" My head and neck hurt, especially the top of my head.

It seems Molly's collar broke as she was flipping around and she "protected" her filly. She butted me in the top of my head as I was bending over looking at the foot. Anthony said I went down like a sack of potatoes and was out like a light—not very original words, but his nonetheless.

Flitter Fry's foot, I discovered later after Molly had acquired a new collar and I had taken a couple of aspirin, had a small quarter crack, which the blacksmith tended to. She was out of training for a few weeks, confined to her stall, and Molly was never happier.

When I stopped doing track work, I stopped seeing goats. I guess I went six or seven years without coming across one, but it really didn't occur to me. I mean, I never woke up in the morning and said anything like, "Well, now it's been 1,217 days since I last saw a goat." I never thought about it. Out of sight, out of mind.

One evening a client called. "Client" is a pretty loose word for this woman. She was a very nice person and owned one horse—a gelding—which I would see maybe twice a year, and then only to vaccinate him. I would also worm and vaccinate her four cats. Carol, the woman, didn't work, per se; she lived in a small cabin on a few acres—maybe eight to ten—and raised most of her own food, which consisted entirely of vegetables. What little income she had was made up of a small monthly alimony check from her ex-husband and from a very inconsistent influx generated by the sale, at various craft fairs and stores, of hand-painted wall plaques. Hand-painted wall plaques have never been considered among the leading industries.

As I said, one evening she called. "Grant," she asked, "do you know anything about goats?" She had acquired a pregnant nanny, she said, for two reasons: to keep Boris, her gelding, company, and to supply milk for her own consumption.

Carol was not a highly profitable client. I earned maybe $50 a year off Boris, but I didn't charge her for her cats' care (I couldn't justify charging too much to a person who probably had no more than $2,500 in annual income), although she often gave me some of her veggies. And I knew I wouldn't charge her for goat care, so this would be a break-even proposition: The income from Boris would be balanced out by the outgo for the cats and the goat.

Two or three weeks later, the nanny delivered her kid. As I said earlier, nothing is as cute as a baby goat, and this one was particularly adorable. I went to check it when it was two days old, and Carol said, "You're going to bill me for this."

"Oh, probably not," I answered. "I'm not really doing anything but looking her over." I told her she was a beautiful baby goat. "I like goats," I added.

When the kid was ten days old, she took her off the nanny and the baby did well. Carol's original plan was to sell her, but at that time I think the going rate for kids was about $15. Still, $15 to Carol was a big hunk of change.

She called one evening. "Come by tomorrow. I have something for you."

Expecting a bag of corn or a half-dozen tomatoes, I went there as I was heading home the next day.

"This is for you," she said, and handed me the kid.

I protested mildly. I reminded her that she had intended to sell her, that her income wasn't so great that she could just throw away $15, which basically was what she was doing by giving me her kid.

"I called Dr. Walter's office yesterday"—Bob Walter is a small-animal vet—"and asked how much it costs to vaccinate and worm a cat. They told me $22. I figured you've saved me hundreds of dollars over the past few years."

So I had a goat. The children were in their early teens and that was good because a goat plays rough. They named her Buddy—not a very feminine name.

Buddy was a great pet except for one thing: We couldn't keep her *in* anything. There are three types of fencing on the farm: plank (mostly), hog wire, and v-mesh wire (one small paddock).

The plank fencing was no challenge at all to Buddy. She got down on her knees and scooted under the bottom plank. The hog wire presented only minor difficulty, and it took her two or three days to figure out how to escape: She *climbed* it, as if it was a ladder. I never saw how she got out of the v-mesh paddock, but she did. Maybe she climbed it, too.

Once out, she wreaked havoc on our landscaping. Every ornamental shrub we had was evidently quite palatable because she ate them all. A small pear tree was especially delectable; she would stand on her hind legs—even jump—to get its leaves.

She apparently didn't like silver maple leaves—she never ate any—but because of the tree's configuration—a fork about three feet up its trunk, then two large, roughly horizontal branches another two to three feet up from there—she would climb it. Goats are natural climbers. We would often find her "baa"-ing pathetically six to eight feet off the ground because getting up was easier than getting back down—a feat she was never able to master without my intervention. (This was a particularly devious tree as far as animals were concerned; a few years later, this was the one from which Fang would fall.)

She loved the dogs, but I'm not sure how much the affection was returned. They romped and raced together, but when Buddy really got excited, she wanted to butt heads. A poor dog's head is no match for a goat's, and the dogs would usually end up running to the house and barking to get in.

We had Buddy—and no landscaping—for slightly more than a year when her mother died. Carol found her that way one morning, and the postmortem exam showed no reason. We didn't know how old she was, so it may have simply been old age. It happens to the best of us (and to the worst of us).

Carol had given up goat's milk quite a while before her goat died, but Boris and the old nanny had been nearly inseparable, and Carol herself was very fond of her. She told me she was going to buy another, but I lied and told her I was concerned about Buddy. Because she couldn't be kept confined, I told her I feared she would go in the road and be hit by a car. (Buddy had never gone within a hundred feet of the road.) I told her I felt Buddy would be a lot safer at her place, located as it was at the end of a dead-end, mile-long lane.

So Buddy went home. Carol had no landscaping to begin with, so nothing was able to be damaged, although her vegetable crops took a beating. Boris accepted Buddy immediately and the three—the horse, the goat, and the woman (oh, yes—and the cats)—are still living happily ever after.

And we have shrubbery again.

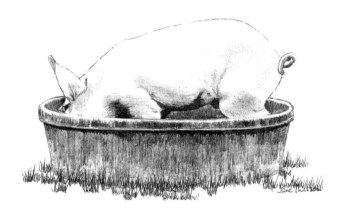

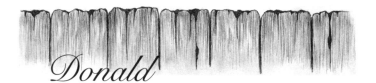

Donald

BEING A HORSE FARM MANAGER is a hard job. Or it should be.

I guess before we go on, the word "manager" as it is used here needs to be defined.

On a large horse farm—and there are those of several thousand acres divided among several tracts, with literally hundreds of horses of all ages—the manager is a person who oversees many assistant managers, who, in turn, may have under them several barn foremen. The manager of one of these huge operations may go months without touching a horse. He is supplied a house and a car, and his salary may be in the six figures.

On the other end of the horse farm spectrum is the five- to ten-acre operation with three to four horses. The owner is a businessman or dentist, or someone else who has a nine-to-five job and can't care for his horses himself (or doesn't want to), so he hires someone to do everything—feed, water, groom, clean stalls, mow, paint fences, paint barns, tease, take the mares to be bred, wash the owner's wife's car, watch the kids for a few minutes while she runs to town, take the dog to the vet, tote that barge, lift that bale, etc. This person is called "manager" in lieu of being given a raise and, believe it or not, it frequently satisfies him. This "manager" must commute to the farm from his own home in his own car, physically works his tail off, and makes very little more than minimum wage.

In between are most farms. Some may have three hundred acres and sixty horses, some twenty-five acres and ten to twelve horses. Some managers may have fifteen to twenty people under them; others have only one. Some managers may have to work with the horses all the time; some work only occasionally.

But whether or not the manager actually cleans stalls and feeds, which can be physically demanding, or directs the operation without any physical contact with the animals, which can be very stressful (I'd much rather clean a barn full of stalls than make sure a crew of six did it right), the position is tough. If it's not done right, there are plenty of others who are willing to try.

Dr. Endor Rzegn, which he pronounced "Ring," owned a big farm. There were a few hundred acres—I never knew how many—and a horse population that hovered right around eighty.

Dr. Rzegn was a computer nerd back before nearly everyone was, and he did things for the government. I never knew what, but he apparently derived substantial income from whatever it was because his farm was beautiful, his house was huge and fancy, and his horses were pretty good—not great, just pretty good.

Mrs. Rzegn dressed well, threw many and great parties (or so I was told—I went to a couple and all I saw were a lot of noisy strangers drinking too much), and drove an extremely expensive foreign sports car. (Dr. Rzegn drove a much more staid and professional foreign luxury car.)

I mention Mrs. Rzegn only because I saw her more often than I saw her husband. She spent a great deal of her free time (which I think is the only kind she had) in her fancy sports car on the roads in the area, and here is where I'd see her. Briefly. She drove so fast and recklessly that all I ever caught was a glimpse of her disappearing in the distance or a blur as she roared past me. On fifty mile an hour narrow county roads where the legal fifty was probably five to ten over reasonable, Mrs. Rzegn drove seventy-five, unless there was a straightaway. Then she'd approach one hundred. She was a terror.

So much for Mrs. Rzegn. Her husband exhibited much better judgment in his driving, and apparently did so in his business, also, because he was, as I said, very successful. His judgment when it came to his horse operation, though, was not as good.

The operation included the entire range of the Thoroughbred sport. He bred his own mares to his own stallions, he raised and raced all his foals, and with rare exception, he brought them all back to the farm at the conclusion of their racing careers. The fillies would become broodmares, and the colts, which he never gelded, would be used as sires if they had been decent runners. If they hadn't, they would be maintained as pensioners, each in his own paddock.

Dr. Rzegn had a farm manager and a crew of five to eight to help the manager. This wasn't enough help, so the manager was a working manager.

Donald was the manager. He was a horse trainer of moderate talent—he would generally get as much effort out of a racehorse as could be gotten—but he was a farm manager of little talent. His heart was on the racetrack for one thing, and for another, he was a little lazy. And rather than hire people who knew how to work on a farm, he hired people from the track. (A horse is a horse, you say, and that's true, but beef is beef, yet you don't hire a cook from a fast-food hamburger stand to be head chef at a four-star restaurant. The jobs are very different.) Another trait of many, perhaps most, horse farm managers is they don't hire anyone who knows more about the job than they do. It is an insecure position, at best.

Everything at Dr. Rzegn's farm, therefore, was done not quite right and not quite completely.

Donald developed a dislike for a horse named Cedar Street through no fault of Cedar Street.

Dr. Rzegn refused to hire a night watchman, so during the foaling season Donald and two of the other employees would share mare-watching duties; one would watch from 6 to 10 P.M., another from 10 to 2 A.M., and the third from

2 to 6, when the workday began. This worked well but no one liked it, especially on cold nights. The 2-to-6 guy *really* disliked it because after sitting up half the night he still had a full day of work ahead of him, so the three would alternate shifts every week or two.

One day after Donald had been on the 2-to-6 shift for several days, he was complaining mightily while I was there checking some mares.

"Gee, Donald," I said, "why don't you ask Dr. Rzegn to install a closed-circuit camera with a microphone. Then you can stay inside in front of a TV screen and if you doze off, the sounds from the mike will wake you."

He loved the idea. Within three days they had the system in and operating. The first mare to foal following installation did so around 11 P.M. Donald saw her lie down and begin on TV, and he got to the barn in two minutes.

The second mare foaled around 3:30 A.M. Donald had gone to sleep around midnight, but he turned the volume way up and the sounds of the mare lying down and grunting woke him. He was there in plenty of time to see her have her foal.

He was happy and his crew was happy. No more drawing straws to see who had to share night duty. "Doc," Donald said to me one day, "this is the greatest thing we ever did here."

A week or so later, though, he began his dislike of Cedar Street.

The mare in the foaling stall that night was Blissful. She was due—maybe past due at 350 days—and she had been under the camera for nearly two weeks. In the stall next to the foaling stall was Maple Street, at 330 days probably not due for at least a week, maybe two.

At about midnight that night, Donald turned up the volume and went to sleep. At about 4:30 he was awakened by thrashing, grunting, and a few weak nickers. He looked at the TV screen. There was Blissful, acting like her name—standing quietly munching on some hay.

The noise continued and Donald watched, but Blissful did nothing. So rather than check to see what was going on, he turned down the volume and went back to sleep for about an hour.

He was awakened again at a quarter to six by a pounding on his door. Max, one of the farmhands, had arrived for work a few minutes early and found

Maple Street, in the stall next to the foaling stall, down and straining. The stall was badly torn up, indicating that she had been at it for quite a while.

I was called, and fortunately I only lived twenty minutes away. Maple Street had a malpresentation—both front legs were bent back at the knees—and because she had been trying for so long, there was no chance to straighten the legs, so we sent her to a clinic where a C-section was performed.

Luck was with us. Both Maple Street and the foal survived, albeit at great expense. Counting surgery, hospitalization, medication, and everything else, it cost Dr. Rzegn about $5,000. Donald caught hell once the story was learned. (Why did he tell it? Who knows.) And he blamed the foal. He sure wasn't going to blame himself.

The foal, a colt that Mrs. Rzegn named (she always named the foals) Cedar Street, was one of those rare babies that loved people. Perhaps it was due to his hospitalization when he received so much attention and had so much human contact, but I've seen some that turned out to hate people as a result of the same situation.

In any event, Cedar Street was thoroughly disliked by Donald, but the reverse was not the case. Cedar Street would rather be with people than with horses. When he and his mom returned to the farm and could be turned out with other mares and foals, he would leave her side and come across the field if he saw a person. When it was time to be brought in to be fed, he was the first one at the gate. And later, after he was weaned, he wouldn't run around and act silly like the other weanlings did when it was time to bring them in. He'd come directly to whomever entered the weanling paddock. (All young horses should be this way.) Frequently, he would linger around the gate in case someone should come by and want a horse to pet.

That fall, after weaning, Donald's dislike for Cedar Street increased. The days were comfortable and the nights were mild, so the horses were put out at night after being fed in their stalls. In the mornings, they were fed in the fields. Most fields had ground feeders (large, untippable nylon tubs), but the two weanling fields had fence feeders (nylon again, but they hung on fence planks).

One morning there was a dense fog, easily the worst I have ever seen in the area. You couldn't see five feet. Feeding the horses with ground feeders was tricky; they couldn't see the person bringing the feed and he couldn't see them. They ran around jockeying for a position at a feeder and could easily run into or over the guy with the bucket of feed.

The two fields with fence feeders were easier and safer. The man could walk along outside the field and place the feed in each feeder, and the horses could sort out among themselves which ate from which feeder and there was no chance that the man dispensing the feed would be damaged.

Donald, being a little lazy and realizing that a chance existed that he could be stepped on or run over if he entered a field full of horses that couldn't see him—and being the boss—chose to feed the horses in the fields with the fence feeders. These were the weanlings.

In a field of six weanling fillies he saw a couple of shapes in the fog and heard hoofbeats. Then he went to the field that held Cedar Street and eight other weanling colts. He went down the fence, scooping feed into the feeders as he came to them. As he passed the gate, there was a weanling silhouetted there in the fog. Horses, especially young ones, are herd animals. Where there is one, there so are the others. Usually. Donald knew this.

The feeding was done between 6 and 6:30 that morning. At about 7:30 the fog still hadn't lifted. Mrs. Rzegn, who wisely chose not to speed through the countryside in the fog, received a phone call from a neighboring farm owner. It seemed that eight weanlings ran into one of his barns. Did they belong to the Rzegns?

Mrs. Rzegn told him she didn't know. She called Donald at the training barn and told him what the neighbor had said. Were they missing any weanlings?

"No, ma'am," he assured her. "I fed the weanlings myself."

The fog lifted around 9. Max drove the manure spreader, and this morning he was going to spread it in the field that held the nine weanlings—Cedar Street's field. Within ten minutes of the time he left the barn, he was back.

"Donald, some of the weanlings are gone! Some planks are down in the back of the field and the only one there is Cedar Street!"

Donald, of course, again caught hell from Dr. Rzegn when he heard the story. Fortunately, the neighbor had put all the loose weanlings in stalls, so except for a few nicks and scratches, all were okay. Donald blamed his lambasting by Dr.

Rzegn on Cedar Street. "That damned horse is too damned stupid to even get away when he has the chance!" he told me one day.

Eventually Cedar Street and the other young horses were broken and put in training. There were fourteen—one had colicked and died as a yearling—and Donald got seven of them to the races as two-year-olds. Cedar Street was one of the seven. This is when Donald was done in and he blamed Cedar Street.

A serious shortcoming in some horse owners is the belief "If I own the horse, it *must* be good." Dr. Rzegn fervently believed this. All of his horses *had* to run in allowance or stakes races; he would not allow any to be put in a claiming race.

Unfortunately, all horses are *not* allowance or stakes class. They have no (or limited) ability and need to run in claiming races if they are going to win anything. (Some can't even win there.) There are class divisions in claiming races, too; a $40,000 claiming race is not far from allowance class, a $2,500 claiming race is not far from the glue factory.

As I said earlier, Donald was an okay trainer. His percentage of winners was low, but that was Dr. Rzegn's fault. Donald wasn't allowed to run the horses at the level they belonged. He had been after Dr. Rzegn for years to let him run those horses that needed it in claiming races. Dr. Rzegn steadfastly refused.

Okay, seven of the two-year-olds from Cedar Street's crop raced at two. Four won—one was a stakes winner—and two placed and looked promising for their three-year-old years. It was an excellent racing season for Dr. Rzegn's stable.

Cedar Street, however, did horribly. He started five times and beat three horses, all three in one race (there were twelve runners). He was *last* four times. Donald told Dr. Rzeng that Cedar Street would never win in decent company, that he needed to be run in claiming races.

"He'll mature as a three-year-old," Dr. Rzegn assured him.

He didn't. In his first two starts at three, Cedar Street ran eighth of ten and ninth of nine. Donald said he either had to be taken out of training or be put in a claiming race.

Dr. Rzegn wouldn't hear of either. After two more starts, in which he was beaten a total of 42 lengths, Donald insisted again that Cedar Street be entered in a claiming race or taken out of training.

"Is he sound?" Dr. Rzegn asked.

"Yes, he's sound!" snapped Donald. "He can't run fast enough to hurt himself!"

I was there for that exchange. Dr. Rzegn didn't like what he heard and the way it was said, but you could see he was wavering on the subject of Cedar Street.

A few days later, Donald told Dr. Rzegn that there was a $7,500 maiden claiming race coming up and he would like to enter Cedar Street in it.

Surprisingly, but grudgingly, Dr. Rzegn consented. Max said he was going to mark this day on the calendar.

On the morning of the race, Dr. Rzegn was pacing back and forth and wringing his hands.

"What's the matter?" Donald naively asked.

"Oh, Donald! We're going to lose Cedar Street," Dr. Rzegn fretted. "Everybody in the world will put in a claim for him."

"Don't worry, Dr. Rzegn," Donald reassured him. "Nobody in his right mind would claim that nickel son of a bitch."

It wasn't the right thing to say. Dr. Rzegn fired him on the spot.

The next—and last—time I saw Donald was about two months later at a Burger King. He was out of work and running out of money.

"That damned horse," he muttered. "That miserable damned horse!"

"What are you talking about?" I asked.

"That damned Cedar Street. Everything's his fault."

Epilogue: Donald was right. No one claimed Cedar Street that day. He ran fifth of twelve, the best race he ever ran. Maybe a drop to $5,000 would have made him a winner, but we'll never know. Dr. Rzegn's new trainer was ordered to return him to allowance races and he ran six more times at three, never beating a horse. Now he's a middle-age pensioner on Dr. Rzegn's farm. Mostly, he stands at his gate, waiting for someone to come by and pet him.

Maple Street, his dam, was not bred the year she had the C-section. She was bred the next year, and the next, and the next, etc., and never got in foal again. This is not an unusual sequel to a C-section in a mare. Dr. Rzegn blamed Donald for this. Donald blamed Cedar Street, of course. Maple Street died at the age of twenty-one; she had not had a foal in nine years.

Dr. Rzegn's refusal to run his horses at the level they needed to be, combined with the failure to introduce new blood into his breeding stock, caused him to eventually go out of the competitive horse business. He still has the farm, but it's filled with pensioners and he keeps two men to take care of them. He reluctantly sold some of his horses, and old age has culled several more. I guess there's about thirty head there now. I still go there three or four times a year to give them the minimal veterinary care they receive.

Mrs. Rzegn missed a curve at about seventy-five one day. Her fancy sports car was totaled and she was nearly so, but she recovered (three months in the hospital) and bought a new, faster fancy sports car.

I heard that Donald finally got a few cheap horses to train for a man in Ohio.

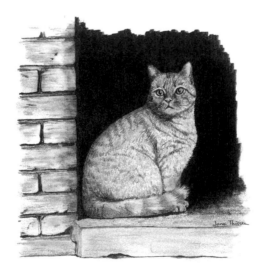

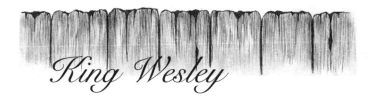

King Wesley

I HAVE ALWAYS WANTED to own a racehorse. To *race* a racehorse. I think anyone who has ever gone to the races or been involved in any way in racing wants to.

But it's expensive and the chances are great—maybe even probable—that it will be a money-losing endeavor. For every Cigar or Secretariat, there are a thousand that don't meet their expenses even if they're winners.

Today it will cost an owner $60 to $150 *a day* just to keep a horse in training. That's what trainers charge, and it doesn't include incidentals like vet, farrier, and vanning bills, which can easily add up to an additional thousand dollars a month. Of course, I wouldn't have to worry about vet bills if I owned a horse and raced him here in Kentucky, but I'm not a trainer and that's the killer expense.

And so much can go wrong. One bad step and all of a sudden you no longer own a racehorse, only a large—and lame—pet. And I think something like only 54 percent of registered Thoroughbreds ever win a race. I don't know (but I should) what percentage of horses earn enough to support themselves, but it's low. Real low.

The odds are definitely against the person who has limited funds, but that didn't and hasn't stopped me from wanting to do it.

Putting all the cons out of my mind, and without discussing it with my wife, I bought a yearling one day with the plan to race him. We had just bought the farm, so it was many years ago, back when I was still doing a lot of track work.

I hadn't planned to buy this yearling. As a horse doctor, I faithfully attend all the local sales because there is always the chance that someone there will need a vet and I can make a buck or two. Also, out-of-state horsemen have at times asked me to bid on horses for them.

This particular sale I had been asked by a man in Pennsylvania to look at a few yearlings for him and give him my opinion. I was there early on the morning of the day they were selling, and while looking at them, I noticed a dark bay colt being groomed by a young woman and I liked his looks. I asked the girl what his number was.

"One-twenty-one," she replied.

I looked him up in the catalogue. It was an amazing pedigree: He was closely inbred.

His sire, King Edward, had been a good racehorse—he had earned more than a half-million dollars—but King Edward's pedigree was borderline and he had not met with great success as a sire. "Moderately useful" is the best that can be said of him.

The colt's dam, Frosty Jan, had been a nice but not outstanding race filly. She had won two races and placed in a couple of cheap stakes, but the interesting part: She was a half sister to King Edward himself.

This made the colt inbred to the dam of King Edward and Frosty Jan, a mare named Lilly Rose, herself a stakes-placed winner. Many pedigree "experts" call this "intense" inbreeding, but it's not. Sure, it's close, but that's all.

People associate inbreeding with mutations, freaks of nature, and lack of vigor because it has been drummed into our heads that the closeness of the genes can bring forth deleterious and detrimental characteristics, but the closeness can just as easily bring forth desirable characteristics. Inbreeding to a good performer may well produce another good performer. I don't know if this colt's breeder had this in mind when he planned the mating or if he just got his wires crossed, but the potential intrigued me.

The colt was very handsome, actually resembling King Edward to a great extent. Maybe, I thought, he would resemble him in performance, too. I called my client in Pennsylvania and reported on the yearlings I had looked at for him, and told him I had seen a very nice colt. Was he interested?

"What's his number?" he asked.

"One-twenty-one."

There was silence on the line for a minute while he apparently looked for number 121 in his catalogue. Finally he spoke again. "Good grief, no. Did you look at that pedigree? There's no telling what you'll end up with."

Which was precisely my point. I decided to be present when he entered the sale ring that afternoon. I wanted to see what he brought.

When his time came, people were pointing at him and laughing. The announcer even made a joke about his pedigree.

The bidding on him was slow. It started at $1,000 after the auctioneer pleaded and went up $200 or $300 a crack as the bids were begged. The auctioneer started to knock him down at $2,500, but I thought it was too cheap. I bid $2,700. Somebody came back at $3,000, so I figured, okay, he's yours.

But then someone else came in at $3,200 and the bidding made another slow, tedious climb, finally reaching $4,700. Once again, the knock-down was coming.

"$5,000. Do I hear $5,000? $5,000?" The hammer was poised.

Someone near me said, "Who in his right mind would pay that much money for *that?*"

That offended me. There was nothing wrong with him or his pedigree. I raised my hand. The bid spotter made his sound—something between a shout and a burp—signifying he saw me, and the hammer fell.

"$5,000," said the auctioneer. "Billy." He nodded toward my spotter. Billy, in turn, nodded at me. I had bought a horse.

When I got home, my wife's less-than-overjoyed response to my announcement was "You did *what!?!*" I sensed displeasure.

A discussion ensued, most of which centered on my lack of responsibility and "money-grows-on-trees" mentality. She pointed out that we had recently committed ourselves to a large mortgage on a farm, that a $20,000 barn was being built in "our backyard," and that I had just bought a $15,000 broodmare eight months earlier in January.

"Where is the money all going to come from?" she asked. It was a reasonable question.

I mumbled something about the veterinary account having enough it in to pay for him (which I had already done), but she reminded me that the veterinary account was merely a stopping-over point for the money we needed for our everyday existence.

She was right, of course. I agreed we'd sell him as a two-year-old in training in the spring sale.

When he arrived at the farm the next day, I found he was a nasty booger, so I gelded him, then turned him over to a woman trainer I knew who agreed to give me a break on her normal rates. Also, I arranged for an exercise rider who owed me a couple hundred dollars I would never see. He was a good rider if not financially solvent.

The now-gelding, which I named King Wesley, was a handful, but he broke and trained uneventfully. One day I asked Bonnie, the trainer, if he looked as if he had any ability.

"No," she answered. "He's just another horse. And hard to work with."

I still wanted to race him, but her opinion made me feel better about the agreement to sell him. Bonnie repeated her opinion later and added she hoped I would get back my initial investment. I didn't relay that to my wife. She would have killed me.

The weekend of the two-year-olds in training sale arrived. By sale rules, the entrants were paired randomly to perform on the track for prospective buyers. King Wesley was a one-horse consignment, and he was assigned to work with (against?) a well-bred colt from a sixteen-horse consignment.

Preston, the exercise rider, asked, "What do you want me to do with him?"

"Just take it easy," I said, "but don't let him be embarrassed."

"I'll talk to the other horse's trainer and see what he plans to do with his horse and I'll just stay with him," Preston suggested.

He came back to see me a half hour later. "He said he just wants the buyers to see how his horses move. He's gonna take it easy, so I'll just keep Wesley alongside him."

The horses went to the track in the designated pairs. The onlookers were betting among themselves as each duo performed.

Finally, Wesley and the other horse came onto the track. A guy standing next to me said to his companion, "Hey, look at this. We got a freak!" He showed him Wesley's pedigree.

His friend laughed. "Who would do something like that?"

The two horses moved around the track to the gate. "Who do you want?" asked the first guy.

"I'll take the freak," chuckled his buddy. "It's only twenty bucks."

Wesley and the other horse entered the gate and a moment later they broke. Preston came out easily on Wesley, but the rider on the other horse was flat down on his mount and whipping him. He zoomed out ten lengths ahead of Wesley and Preston.

Preston sat down on Wesley and began to ride him. He gained on the other colt, but that horse's rider was really getting into him. With about a sixteenth mile of the three furlongs left, Wesley caught him. By the end he was a length ahead and pulling away. His time turned out to be the fastest of the entire sale.

I went back to the barn where Preston was fuming. "Son of a bitch said he was gonna take it easy. I coulda aired if I'da known." He mumbled on about anal apertures and "nobody makes *my* horse look bad."

The next day, Wesley sold for $12,000. After expenses, I made about $4,000 profit.

Bonnie had been wrong about his price and wrong about his ability, too. Later that summer, he made his debut in a $12,500 maiden claimer and won easily. A couple of starts later he won for $15,000 and was claimed. He eventually won several allowance races and even ran in a couple of stakes but ran in the middle of the pack each time. He finally settled in as about a $35,000 to $40,000 claimer and distance didn't matter—long, short, or in between, it was all the same to Wesley. He was probably claimed five or six times over the years. He never took a bad step and remained sound through the age of five. In those four years he earned about $130,000.

I sure wish we'd have kept him.

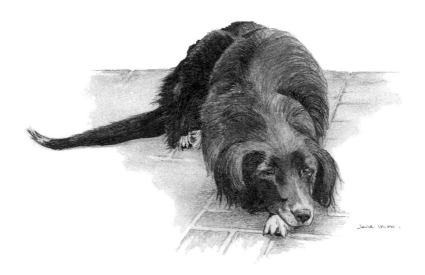

PART TWO

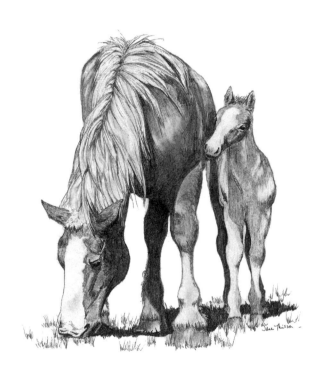

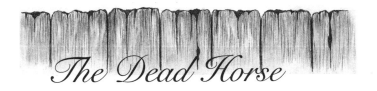

The Dead Horse

I AM NOT A BELIEVER in Fate or Destiny. I don't think things are predestined or somehow predetermined somewhere in the Great Cosmos; I believe we make our own destinies, that our fates are in our own hands. Occasionally though, an incident will occur that makes me wonder just a little.

"My trainer tells me again he's the best I've ever had, the best he's ever trained," my Jamaican friend told me over the phone. "He says he doesn't know how good he can be."

Pretty encouraging words for a "dead" horse.

Quite often, Thoroughbred racehorses are named after living people. The Jockey Club, the registration body of the Thoroughbred world, allows this only if the person gives written permission—*if* the person's actual name is used.

I have no idea how many horses have been named for people. If the horse turns out to be a good one, we hear about it, but if the horse can't or won't run, or is in some way prevented from running, the origin of a name, or even the name itself, is never learned.

Some horses have been named for people without using the person's name, per se. Arpee Fore, for instance, a decent stakes winner several years back, was named for Richard Perry, IV (R. P. 4), his breeder and a close friend of the person who bought the colt as a yearling. The great Kelso was named after a friend of his owner. My Jamaican friend once named a filly after his four daughters: Laura, Kim, Michelle, and Karen. The name: La Kimika. (Students of French searched vainly for a translation.) Another friend named a filly Mary Beth, after his girlfriend. Names such as these don't need written permission, but had he used his girlfriend's full name—Mary Beth Peters—it would have been necessary.

Several years ago, there was a Sinatra. One must assume permission was required for that. Unfortunately, he never amounted to anything (I believe an injury prevented his racing). I assume, too, that Paul Hornung, a useful but unremarkable runner that performed shortly after the football player of the same name retired, and Bobby Powers, whoever he is (was), also needed permissions. There are dozens.

Veterinarians have occasionally had horses named for them. I'm not sure why—maybe it's in lieu of paying the vet bills. I remember a couple: Beauchamp and Dr. Mercer, both pretty good performers. I don't know how many others there have been, but I do know of at least one.

Many years ago I boarded several mares for my friend who lives in Jamaica. They weren't great mares, but they generally produced runners that paid their way, and because he raced them rather than sold them, that was what he wanted.

An explanation, which will prove to be lengthy, I fear, is necessary here for those not familiar with the vagaries of marketing Thoroughbreds. There are "fashionable" and "unfashionable" pedigrees, and in many cases these are very subjective calls. A "fashionable" pedigree consists of highly recognizable names of highly successful horses. An "unfashionable" pedigree, therefore, is made up of totally unrecognizable names of totally unsuccessful horses. There are, of course, many steps in between, leading to the absolute subjectivity of any assessment.

At the upper end of this scale—the supremely fashionable pedigrees—are those mares whose offspring command top dollar at the annual yearling sales. Real people can't afford these horses, but the best chances of acquiring a superior racehorse lie here. And of course, at the lower end—where the yearlings sell for a few hundred dollars—the chances of getting anything but a hay-eating liability are practically nil.

In the upper regions of the vast in-between area lie pedigrees that repeatedly produce racehorses that pay their way and make money for their owners, but rarely seem to come up with a great horse, although lightning occasionally strikes and a super runner appears. If you're selling from these pedigrees, you'll do well but you'll never get rich. If you're buying from these pedigrees, you need deep but not bottomless pockets and you have a good chance of getting a racehorse that will be both fun and profitable to own.

If, however, you *own* this type of pedigree *and* race the offspring, you do not have to buy a potential racehorse and you still have the opportunity for a profitable venture onto the racetrack. These were the type of mares my friend owned and I boarded for him.

Okay, back to the story.

Among these mares was one named Princess of Kali (wherever that is). At the time we are considering here, she was seventeen years old and had produced eight foals of racing age. Two of them never made it to the track, but of the six that did, five had done very well, each having earnings of around $100,000, plus or minus five grand or so. One had even won a couple of small stakes.

Princess, though, was on the verge of becoming someone else's mare. She had not gotten in foal for two straight years, and even though she was pregnant now, her owner was leaning heavily toward selling her after she foaled. This practice is fairly common when an older mare begins to lose fertility because, even though she stops producing foals, she continues to pile up board and vet bills.

Why would someone buy an older mare with a reproductive problem? you ask. Hope, the *raison d'etre* of the horse-racing world—hope that she *will* get in foal for you and will once again produce one of those hundred-thousand-dollar earners. Plus the fact that, even though she is a cull, she still upgrades someone else's mares, someone who has a little less-fashionable mares than the seller. It works down like this until the bottom is reached, where there are no less-fashionable or successful mares. But there's a market even for these, too; unfortunately, it's the dog food companies.

I wasn't crazy about this plan of selling Princess. Princess was a beautiful mare, but more importantly, she was a real sweetheart—gentle and kind and easy to work with. And so were her foals. (I'd a whole lot rather have a good agreeable horse than a great nasty one if I have to work with it myself.) Even *more* important, however, was the fact that I was paid to board Princess, and if she was sold that would no longer be the case. Boarders—good-paying boarders—are hard to come by in the horse business and no one wants to lose one.

But my friend was partial to Princess, and she was in foal to a stallion he *really* liked. He had originally planned to sell her if she conceived to this particular stallion, an English horse named Chadwick Forest, but the more he thought about it, the more he wanted that foal she was carrying, so she got at least a temporary reprieve.

"Let's get the foal," he told me, "then we can breed her back and sell her next fall."

Reluctantly I had agreed, but she wasn't my mare, so my opinion carried little weight. (If any.)

Adding to his thinking on selling Princess was the fact that she had not gotten in foal early this time. After two years of nonproduction, it had still been necessary to breed her to Chadwick Forest *five* times before she conceived. At seventeen, it did not bode well for the future.

Even at that, her foaling date should be a not-too-bad April 20 or so, and April is the month in which most foals arrive each year. A potential problem, however, was the fact that, for reasons I don't fully understand, older mares, especially older mares that haven't been in foal for a while, often carry their foals longer than the calculated time, sometimes a *lot* longer.

For this reason, I was not alarmed or concerned when mid-April came and Princess wasn't showing any signs of impending parturition: no bag filling, no vulvar relaxation, etc. In the previous pregnancies she had been through with me, she had progressed normally and given ample forewarning, so I had no qualms about leaving her out in the pasture on the night of April 17.

Unexpectedly—at least I hadn't expected it—it rained cats and dogs that night. The day had been sunny and around 70 degrees, but by morning, in addition to the downpour, the temperature had dropped to nearly 40 degrees. It was miserable, not fit for man nor beast, and certainly not fit for foaling.

Early in the morning—5:20 A.M., to be exact—Laurie called and said she would be late—her boyfriend's car wouldn't start (for the third time in a month), and she had to take him to work (again)—so I went forth to tend to the horses before I began my veterinary calls. This was my busiest time of the year by far—twelve- to sixteen-hour days—and I really didn't have the time to lose, but the horses had to be fed. As I sloshed toward the barn, I found myself hoping the boyfriend would get his car fixed properly, and soon.

All the horses, except two mares with week-old foals, had been left out overnight. A 50-degree low with no rain had been anticipated and that certainly wasn't too cold for horses, and horses that stay outside at night don't have stalls that need to be cleaned the next day. But this weather was awful, and I had to bring them all in so they could dry off and warm up. I began with the mares with foals, so the mares that had not yet foaled and the two mares that were not in foal were last. All the horses were saturated and shivering badly.

The rain had lessened somewhat as I finally headed for the field Princess shared with two other pregnant mares, both due to foal in late May. One of these was a screwball named Lucky Florian, also owned by my friend. It took nothing to make Florian flip out. A scrap of paper wafting by on a breeze would nearly bring on apoplexy. Sudden noises, a strange vehicle pulling up to the barn, Gladys the goose coming to the barn for her corn—any of these or a dozen other things would cause Florian to prick her ears, flare her nostrils and snort, become bug-eyed, raise her tail, and run in circles, whether or not she was being led. She was a barrel of laughs. I didn't hate her, but if a mare was going to be sold, I wished she would be the one.

On this particular morning as I entered the field, Florian was running in circles. I figured it must be the rain; she had been rained on before—only four or five days earlier, in fact—but with her mind it was possible she didn't remember it.

But then I saw Princess. She was lying flat on her side and behind her was a large brown blob. I ran to her. She was alive but exhausted. The blob behind her was a foal. At first I thought it was dead, but when I got closer I saw it (I didn't bother to check to see if it was a he or a she at that point) was also alive, but barely.

Florian was running circles around us as I tried to get Princess up. I stopped and caught the idiot and put her in the barn, where she could run her circles in a twelve-by-twelve stall. Then I went to the house to get my wife—I needed help with Princess—and to get a dry jacket. By this time I was as wet as the horses and shivering just as they were. I made a mental note to suggest to Laurie that she either get her boyfriend a new car or get a new boyfriend.

We were able to get Princess up with much difficulty, but the foal was something else. Because of the rain, I couldn't tell how long he had lain there, but it must have been a while (a wet foal usually means it's only been a matter of minutes); it was only able to blink weakly and gasp. There was no way it was going to get to the barn by itself, so I picked it up and carried it.

My wife, who had seen many foals over the years and who was *never* pessimistic, took one look at the miserable little wretch and said, "It will never live." I was sure she was right.

Unfortunately, it was a big foal—120 pounds anyway—and equally, or more, unfortunately, it was at least 150 feet from where we were in the field to the barn. I wasn't sure I could carry it that far.

But we got there. The foal, which from this point I will refer to as "he" because I checked when we got in a stall, still did nothing but gasp and blink. I called a van company and requested the equine ambulance as fast as it could get here. Then I called a vet clinic that had a neonatal intensive care unit and told them I was sending in a critical foal. "I hope he'll still be alive when he gets there," I added.

While we waited, we thawed some colostrum that we keep on hand. While attempting to pass a nasogastric tube so we could feed it to the foal, the kids came in the barn, announcing they had missed their bus and would, therefore, be late for school. I made another mental note: introduce Laurie to some young men with new (and reliable) cars.

The colt spent ten days in the neonatal unit at a cost of nearly $7,000. Initially the vets at the clinic told me they were sure he was going to die, but by his fourth day he was able to stand with help, so I arranged for a nurse mare because Princess never developed any milk.

When he and his adopted mother came back to the farm, he was basically just another foal, albeit a lot weaker than the older babies, so we did not turn him out with them. Lucky Florian and the other mare both foaled on the same evening three weeks later, so I put him with these two little guys; normally, I wouldn't put a month-old foal with foals this young, but all three were at about the same strength level. By weaning time, he had developed to a point to where it couldn't be told that he had ever been at death's door, and by the time he left the farm late in his yearling year to be broken and trained, he had actually advanced well beyond the other foals of his crop. He was big and beautiful and had his birth mother's wonderful disposition.

Princess, in the meantime, responded to TLC and was bred back in late May but didn't conceive. The decision was made to keep her, but when she didn't conceive the next year, either, my friend told me to find a good home for her. We gave her to a friend of Laurie, who got a foal from her three years later, when she was twenty-one (Princess, not Laurie's friend).

Lucky Florian's foal, also a colt, had his mother's outlook and idiocy. For the year and a half he was on the farm, he acted as if he had never seen a stall in his life whenever he was put inside one, which was daily. He jumped every time he saw a muck basket, which was also daily, and he was scared to death of Cat, Gladys, and the ducks, whom he also saw daily. Those of us who have mundane, routine lives should envy him; to him, nothing was ever mundane or routine—everything he ever saw or did was totally new to him. And terribly frightening.

Laurie didn't get a new boyfriend despite my hopes, but the old boyfriend eventually got another, but not new, car. It was far more reliable and that problem was resolved.

Although I told the whole story to my friend and made certain he knew that it was the ICU that saved his colt's life, and indeed, it was my carelessness in not watching a mare that was due to foal that created the problem in the first place, he gave me full credit for saving the foal. He asked if he could have the "honor" of naming the colt after me: Dr. Kendall. (I suggested the name Brain Dead for Lucky Florian's colt, but he chose the original Florian's Luck for him.)

Dr. Kendall broke and trained brilliantly. Nigel turned down $50,000 for him, then $80,000, then *$100,000!* This brings us back to the quote with which we began this tale, where he called me from Jamaica to rave on Dr. Kendall's progress.

It was early October of Dr. Kendall's two-year-old year when that call came. He said the trainer had a race picked out for "next week" and Dr. Kendall would make his first start, and "he tells me he will win it by ten lengths!" He said he would bet fifty across the board for me.

I knew Nigel's trainer, a middle-aged gentleman named Derrick O'Rourke, was not given to exaggeration or even enthusiasm about the horses in his care. I had never seen Derrick excited about any horse he had trained, and he had had some very good ones over the years; for him to flat-out state that Dr. Kendall would "win it by ten lengths" was tantamount to a sure thing. If the colt was half as good as Derrick was promoting him to be, I—or my name—was going to be famous, at least around the racetracks.

Five days later, my wife came to the barn to get me. "Nigel just called," she said, "and he wants to talk to you right away."

Anticipating that this was the news that Dr. Kendall had made his start and won easily as expected, I went immediately to the house and called.

"Oh, my boy," he said when I reached him, "Dr. Kendall went to the track this morning to exercise prior to his race tomorrow. He dropped dead. They tell me it was a heart attack."

❦

I don't know if his death was Fate—after all, maybe he was supposed to have died two years earlier in that cold April rain—but I guess being a racehorse was not his destiny.

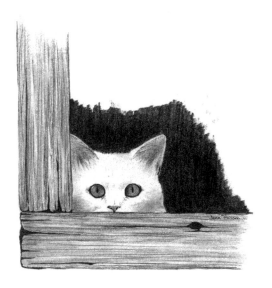

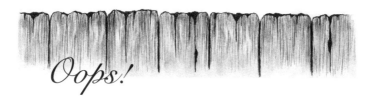

Oops!

SOMETIMES WE (VETERINARIANS) MAKE MISTAKES. Or at least, I hope that's a "we"; I know I make plenty and I hope I'm not the only one goofing up.

Mistakes range from saying the wrong thing to doing the wrong thing, from inconsequential to fatal, and I've made them all, I'm sorry to say. I'm happy to say, though, to the best of my knowledge, I've made only one fatal mistake. It was one too many, of course, and I lost sleep over it for quite a while.

A two-year-old filly died because of me. As bad as it was, it was made worse by the fact that another vet owned her. He lived in another state and sent her here to board at a farm where I did the work. She was to be bred.

I protested when I learned that. I knew the guy, so I called him and questioned his decision. A two-year-old filly is perhaps like a thirteen-year-old girl: All the parts are there and usually functional, and the urge is there, but the maturity is not. I'm not referring only to physical maturity—just as a thirteen-year-old girl has considerable physical development remaining, so does a two-year-old filly— there is also the question of mental (emotional?) maturity. Even though the two-year-old filly will be three when she foals, she is no more ready for mother-hood than the thirteen-year-old girl who will probably be fourteen at the time of delivery.

It's a bad idea—both horsewise and humanwise—yet it's done. Fortunately, it's not a widespread problem in horses, but even one is too many.

This filly in question had been injured in training in November of her yearling year, so her racing career never began. She had been particularly hard to handle, and her own attitude led to her injury. And to her demise.

A little maturity, though, may have helped everything. Had they quit on her instead of fighting with her, the training injury may never have occurred. Six months more of handling and gentling may have made a big difference. This is only conjecture, of course, but patience is an important part of horsemanship, and I think this comes under the general heading of "patience."

Likewise in her breeding. Had they let her mature during her two-year-old year she may well have been more amenable at three to what we needed to do to prepare her for breeding. And, too, she would have been more physically mature, but greed enters into the horse business and this was motivated by greed: The sooner she can be raced and bred, the sooner there might be a financial return.

As I said, I called the vet owner of this two-year-old filly, named Spinning Wheel. "All she's done is cost me money," he complained. "She needs to start paying some back!" He further explained that she was his filly and it was his decision and really none of my business. After our conversation, I hoped he didn't have any daughters.

Spinning Wheel had arrived at my client's farm in mid-January. She fought the teaser steadily 'til late February, so my client asked me to check her to be sure she had a reproductive tract that was functional. A filly that age may still have immature ovaries, and indeed, some adult mares have infantile reproductive tracts and can never be bred. Also, it was winter and many mares just don't cycle during winter.

To determine the size of her ovaries and uterus, it was necessary to palpate her. This procedure rarely makes mares' Top Ten List of Things They Most Enjoy, but fortunately 99+ percent of them tolerate it very well.

But there is that one-half percent or so that just plain don't like to be palpated, and as the procedure must of necessity be done from the rear end of the mare, they have ways of showing their disapproval so that there is little question as to what they're trying to tell you.

The first time I attempted to palpate Spinning Wheel she raised such heavy objections, even with tranquilization, that I chose to try again later, maybe in a few weeks. My client reported to her vet owner that Spinning Wheel may end up being a problem, but the owner complained about the board bill and told my client to tell me to try again sooner.

So around the first of March I did, under protest. I wanted to wait until perhaps mid-April, when the weather was a little warmer and the days were a little longer, and most importantly, the filly was a little older.

Even under tranquilization, she still would not stand well (as before) and she still attempted to kick (as before), but this time I got my hand in her rectum. The kicking stopped because now she was straining so hard to expel my hand that the kicking apparatus couldn't function.

The rectal wall of a horse is very thin and weak. It is easily perforated. Any time a palpation is performed, the very real danger exists that the palpater's hand will penetrate the rectal wall, allowing fecal matter to enter the peritoneal cavity.

And horses are probably the species most susceptible to fatal peritonitis. Feces, of course, is loaded with bacteria.

Spinning Wheel was straining so hard I knew I had to retract my hand or damage would be done, but I wasn't quick enough. I felt the rectal wall give.

When I pulled out my hand, there was blood on the plastic palpation sleeve. While polluting the air with language I shouldn't use, most of which was directed toward the filly's owner, I gave her a large injection of penicillin, then I called an equine surgery clinic and told them a filly with a rectal tear was on her way.

The farm was way out, so the equine ambulance didn't arrive for nearly forty-five minutes. Spinning Wheel did not load well (we didn't know that before), and it took a half hour to get her on it, then it was forty-five more minutes to the clinic.

The vet there, one of the top surgeons in the area, was ready for her when we arrived. He found the tear and corrected it, and she was placed on a very high level of antibiotics, but peritonitis had already set in and would not be controlled. She died two days later.

Even though we all knew the cause of death, a postmortem exam is always essential when a horse dies, especially in the case of an absentee owner. We are lucky here in central Kentucky to have some outstanding veterinary pathologists; I asked the one doing Spinning Wheel's post to look at her uterus and ovaries while he was in there.

They were very small, he reported to me. In his opinion, it was unlikely that she was breedable at that time.

But I think she would have been—maybe in May, surely the next year. I shouldn't have palpated (obviously), and I should have gotten my hand out sooner when she began straining, but I did and I didn't and I tore through her rectal wall and she died, and I was almost afraid to palpate any mare for quite a while.

Fortunately, none of my other mistakes were quite so costly.

I try to limit my practice to horses. My business card clearly says "Practice Limited to Horses." My Yellow Pages listing says the same thing.

But I can't do it. Some guys can—or claim they can—but I don't know how. With one or two exceptions, my horse-owning clients own other species of animals: dogs and cats mostly; but quite a few also have cattle, and the occasional sheep appears. I have a friend who breeds, raises, and shows Mastiffs, and she is always getting me to do something or another to her dogs. (Mastiffs may be as big as horses, but that's where the similarity ends.)

My horse clients know I'm not equipped to work on other species—different drugs and tools are necessary and I just don't have them—so they don't routinely ask me tend to their nonhorse critters, but there are times when the need arises when I'm there.

At one client's farm one day, a cow was attempting to deliver a calf with a singular lack of success, so I intervened. The calf's head was turned back; it took a little effort to straighten it, but I did and we got the calf into the world. Had I not been there at the time, my client would have called his regular cattle vet but I *was* there, so it was no big deal.

A nonhorse person had a cow problem once and I went to his farm. It was the last operating dairy in this area, and it was on the Fourth of July. The man came to my house, asked if I was the vet, and said he had a cow with a problem. I told him that I didn't work on cows, but he said it was a serious problem and he could not get hold of either of the two cow vets in the area; neither answered the phone. "She's bleedin' bad, Doc," he said. "Please see if you can help her."

Well, as you know, I don't like cows, but I couldn't let one bleed, so I had to go. I followed him to his dairy, and sure enough, she was bleeding badly. She had hooked her milk vein on something and the blood was flowing out in a steady stream. The milk vein is the extremely large vein that runs from the mammary glands along the lower portion of a cow's belly; in some cases, it's as big around as your thumb. I asked him how long she had been bleeding.

"Since this mornin'. She ran into a loose nail when we were bringin' 'em in to milk 'em."

It was after 3 P.M. now. The poor thing had been bleeding for maybe eight or nine hours. It was a wonder she had not bled out and died.

It was obvious it had to be sutured. I approached the cow, but she was very agitated and wouldn't stand still, so I decided I had to tranquilize her. As I was getting the tranquilizer, I noticed that the bleeding was slowing slightly. The dairy farmer also noticed it. "Maybe it's stoppin', Doc."

That's what I was afraid of. The only reason it would stop was if there was no more to come out. Still, I gave her the tranquilizer and got my suturing equipment out of the car.

When I returned to the cow with it, she was dead. All the blood was gone from her circulatory system. In other words, she had bled to death.

The farmer said only, "I'll be damned. How much do I owe you, Doc?"

"Nothing," I replied, and left. Later I learned that he told several people that all day the cow was alive and well and I came and gave her one shot and it killed her.

Several of my clients own those funny-looking little cattle dogs—Australian Shepherds or something like that. These dogs have a tremendously developed herding instinct, but most are well controlled by their owners. Some, however, are always nipping at the heels of the horses trying to get them to go somewhere, whether or not the people involved want them to.

It's aggravating as the dickens to everyone concerned, especially the horses. They kick at the pestiferous little snapping dogs. It makes me so angry that often I find I'm hoping the horse makes contact, but I've never seen it happen. And as I'm back there with the dogs, trying to spec or palp, I find it very inconvenient, scary even. These dogs may be a great idea on a cattle or sheep operation, but they just don't belong on a horse farm.

Be that as it may, there was one of these little dogs that was extremely pesky. One day he was trying to herd a mare I was working on, even though we had her exactly where she needed to be. The mare kicked at the dog, which very gracefully avoided the foot, but he had gotten too close to the edge of the stall door and in darting out of the way he ran into it. The hinge was old and had somehow developed a sharp edge and when he hit it, he received a pretty good gash on his hip.

It needed to be sutured and I was there, so I sutured it. All in all, it was satisfying. I had to sedate the little twerp to work on him, and for the remainder of the time I was there that day—close to an hour—he was not a problem. Unfortunately, he was his old yappy, snappy self the next day.

I carry dog and cat vaccines and wormers for my horse clients' animals. In many cases, these pets are strictly farm animals and would never see a vet other than me, and they need these things. If I charge at all it's only my cost, so this is not a large contributor to my practice income or my family's welfare.

Cats, especially, are frequently neglected on farms. Oh, they're usually fed, but vaccinations and reproductive control are ignored. In order to help keep the kitten population down, I will neuter tom cats belonging to my clients. I'm not equipped to spay the females, but gelding a tom is very easy and quick and inexpensive. Again, I often don't charge for it and if I do, the fee is only for my cost in drugs and supplies.

Several pages ago you were expecting to read of mistakes I'd made, but by now you think I've gotten pretty far afield. We'll call all these intervening pages an introduction and now we're there—to not one but *three* errors.

Crescent Moon Farm had a serious mouse and rat problem in its three barns, so management decided to acquire a cat for each barn. I suggested that they get them from the local animal shelter because they would be vaccinated and neutered already, but that was vetoed because animal shelter cats cost $39 each. The cheapest mare on Crescent Moon was probably worth $100,000, and I couldn't see how $120 for cats would even be noticed, but apparently the person who signed the checks saw it differently.

They decided to check the newspaper and get three free kittens. I suggested they get males because I could geld them and eliminate the problem of kittens in the future. Dan, the farm manager, said he would be certain they were males.

The task of kitten acquisition was assigned to the farm secretary. She took an afternoon off and visited several places that had advertised free kittens, but returned empty-handed. "I can't tell the boys from the girls," she explained.

The next morning Dan went, but returned at noon with the same story. "Some of them look like males, but I'm not sure," he told me when I was there that afternoon to look at a couple of mares. "And the owners aren't sure, either."

"Gee, Dan, if you'd get 'em from the animal shelter there wouldn't be a problem," I said.

He shook his head. "They won't let me spend that much. Will you come with me and tell me which are boys?"

I think you now know where this is heading, but before I continue, let me say that telling a six-week-old boy cat from a six-week-old girl cat is hard and is not an area in which I'm proficient. Still, with a fifty-fifty chance, you'd think I would have selected *one* boy at least, but I didn't. We didn't realize this, however, until they were five or six months old and I tried to neuter them, so instead of $39 each at the animal shelter, Crescent Moon Farm paid my small-animal vet friend $85 each to spay them.

There are two lessons here, one involving cheapness and one involving me, although I'm not sure what it is.

The farm crew had a lot of fun over this for quite a while. I'd be preparing to palp a mare and a groom would raise the tail and say something like, "Just wanna be sure it's a mare, Doc. I know it's confusing." Or a foal would be born and I'd check its sex and the foaling man would say, "Whatever Doc says it is, I'm bettin' the other way."

And there were cruder remarks from time to time, like when someone would ask how I ever had kids and was I sure that one was a boy and the other a girl or did I just choose arbitrarily. I told them that my wife had an anatomy book and checked them out in there before we decided.

If I went into detail on each error I've made through the years, this book would be longer than *War and Peace,* so one more will suffice and then I'll go back to telling you how good I am.

One of the hard, cold, incontrovertible, etched-in-stone facts we learned in vet school is: Horses *cannot* vomit. There is a band of smooth muscle around the esophagus just as it enters the stomach and peristalsis (the movement necessary to propel material through the digestive tract) can't run backward through smooth muscle. Therefore, when something is swallowed, it enters the stomach and can only leave via the small intestine. The only time a horse will regurgitate is at or near the time of death (I should know why, but I don't), and this was indelibly imprinted in our minds by continual repetition by almost every teacher we had in equine clinic. In essence, we were led to believe that there are *three* sure things in this life: death, taxes, and horses don't barf and live to tell about it.

Brenda Bebop was an older mare—in her late teens. She had been money in the bank for years; several of her foals had been stakes winners, one a near-champion. She was very valuable and she was carrying a foal with a $50,000 stud fee.

Her foaling date was nearing but not imminent. Mack, the farm manager, had season tickets to the University of Kentucky basketball games—a religion in this part of the country—but he wouldn't go if he expected a mare to foal the night of a game.

Brenda was only 334 days, and older mares often go a little long, plus her bag wasn't a foaling bag yet, *plus* the University of Tennessee was in town playing UK. There are bigger rivalries than Tennessee-Kentucky, but not many and certainly not around here.

Well, of course, what happened is obvious: Brenda attempted to foal. When it became apparent to the night watchman, a new employee I hadn't met before, that she wasn't going to accomplish it without help, he called me as Mack had instructed him to do.

She had been in labor nearly an hour by the time I got there. That's a *long* time for a mare and I feared that the foal was already dead. Brenda herself was just lying there, flat out and glassy-eyed with no contractions and very little of anything else.

The foal's legs were bent back at the knees. Because there were no uterine contractions and because the foal offered no resistance at all, I was able to straighten the legs relatively easily. As I was doing it, I said, "I'm afraid this little guy's probably dead."

The night watchman made no comment.

Once I had the legs straight, I had him help me pull out the foal. Without the mare's pushing, that's *hard*, but we got him.

The foal just lay there. "He must be gone," I said.

I went to get my stethoscope and when I got back I saw an eye blink. He was alive and with a little rubbing and pounding he perked up somewhat.

Brenda, in the meantime, hadn't moved. We dragged the foal around in front of her, hoping she would rouse when she saw and smelled him, but she didn't.

Then she moved. She stretched her head straight out on the bedding, wretched once, and made a hollow, belching sound. Then a brownish-green, foul-smelling efflux oozed from her mouth. In other words, she vomited.

"Oh, man," I said dejectedly, "she's gonna die."

A moment later, though, she rolled up on her sternum and sniffed her foal. Then she licked him.

Then she stood up, shook herself, and continued to attend to her baby.

Within an hour, the foal got up and nursed. Everything was normal and you'd never know there had been a problem.

The night watchman had said very little the whole time. In fact, I still didn't know his name. I felt him looking at me, so I looked over at him.

"When's she gonna die?" he asked.

About this time, Mack, the farm manager, returned from the basketball game and burst into the barn frantically when he saw my car there. He calmed down considerably when he saw Brenda and her colt standing there, apparently none the worse for the experience. I explained to him what had transpired and went to my car to put things away and prepare to leave.

I heard the night watchman whisper to Mack, "What do you know about this here vet?"

"Why?" asked Mack.

"Well, he said the foal was dead and he ain't," he whispered.

Mack didn't reply.

"And he said the mare was gonna die and she ain't dead. Does he know what he's doin'?"

Even though it seemed at that moment that I had made a mistake, I was actually right. Brenda Bebop *did* die—six years and four foals later. Of old age.

I guess that takes us back to only two sure things: death and taxes.

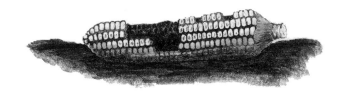

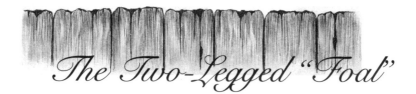

The Two-Legged "Foal"

CERTAIN THOROUGHBREDS, AS I HAVE NOTED before, are said to have the "Look of Eagles." None, however, have ever been described as having the eyesight of eagles.

They, and all horses, don't see well.

In the wild, horses are the hunted and as such have a keenly developed sense of smell. The scent of a far-off predator can be readily picked up if the wind is right. But because a predator may be downwind, horses do have some distance vision.

Their eyes are positioned on the sides of the head, so anything directly in front of them is not seen. This eye positioning, however, enables them to see to each side and even behind them, to a fair extent.

A downwind lion (tiger, leopard, jaguar, whatever) can stand in this field of vision forever, though, and remain unnoticed by the horse, which will acknowledge it only if it moves. I guess, then, the predator itself isn't really seen; only the motion is.

One of the main ways in which people working with horses are hurt is a result of this vision limitation. Something—a dog, a blowing leaf, sometimes only a misinterpreted shadow—appears when a horse is being handled, the horse spooks and jumps, and the handler is stomped. Usually a toe is involved. Bruised and broken toes may actually be the norm among horse farm employees.

And some things are pretty scary to some particular horses. Our seldom-used farm truck was parked in the same spot by the barn every day. One filly, from the day she was born, walked in and out of the barn two to four times a day (depending on whether she would stay in at night or be put out), passing the truck each time. She was eighteen months old when she left us and each time she passed the truck for all those months—and she was never within twenty feet of it—she jumped. One day I tried to lead her over to it so she could see that it was not going to harm her, but she knew better. She would not go anywhere near that killer machine.

We'll get back to horse vision in a minute.

Someone once did a survey and determined that most mares—something like 60 to 70 percent, I think it was—foal between 10 P.M. and 2 A.M. My practice doesn't bear this out, however. I haven't compiled the statistics and I don't intend to, but I'm pretty sure that at least half the mares I have tended over the years have foaled between 3 and 6 A.M. and another 20 to 30 percent—bless them—deliver in the daytime or early evening.

I've had a few clients who called me for every foaling. I'm an early riser anyhow so it never bothered me (much) and I got to charge for it, so I certainly didn't discourage them from doing so. Most, however, call for only two reasons: (1) a problem, or (2) a mare carrying a particularly valuable foal.

One morning several years ago I received a call that was a combination of (1) and (2). A mare named The Queen's Boots was a stakes winner and stakes producer and was carrying a foal from the first crop of a former champion. The farm manager, an excellent horseman of long experience named Bill, had told me he would call at the first signs of Bootsie's parturition. She was somewhere in the 340 to 345–day range when he told me that, so I was expecting the call any day.

About 3:30 A.M. this late April morning in question Bill called. "Bootsie's starting," he said, and I headed for the farm. It took me about a half hour to get there and when I arrived, Bill looked concerned. "She's down and straining," he said, "but nothing's coming."

I stuck my hand in her vagina about an inch and felt the unruptured placenta, but the pressure she was exerting was so great that I could not feel the foal itself to determine position. In response to my hand, Bootsie strained and pushed harder, expelling my hand and ballooning the placenta a few inches through her vulva. Then she got up.

"This has to go," I said, indicating the protruding placenta. Bill was holding her tail; I reached over, plucked the ballpoint pen from his shirt pocket, and poked it into the bloated sack. (A ballpoint works great for this purpose.)

The placenta ruptured and then some. The amount of pressure within it caused by the mare's straining was suddenly released, and placental fluid spewed everywhere—but mostly on Bill. I received some on me, but poor Bill got it full in the face and chest, drenching him. (Anticipating this copious flow, I had stuck the pen into the bag on the side away from me. I'm not as dumb as I look.)

Now able to determine what was amiss, I found that the foal's head was coming ears first instead of nose first, but luck allowed me to reposition it easily and the little guy popped on out. Bootsie was standing and Bill caught the foal—he was already a mess so a little more juice wouldn't matter—and eased it down to the stall floor.

The night watchman was holding Boots and he turned her around so she could see what was going on. Bill and I were attending to her foal—it was a colt—and she stuck her head down to see what she had, but got only as far as Bill.

This was the scent she was searching for! She nuzzled him, she nickered to him. She *licked* him!

He pushed her away but she came right back. She started to paw at him but the guy with the shank pulled her away. This upset her! She jerked him back to Bill and nuzzled and nickered some more.

We finished working on and checking the foal and stepped away from him, knowing that Bootsie would recognize her error when she saw him. But she didn't. She ignored the colt and went to Bill.

"Let's leave the stall," I suggested, "so she can figure out what she has."

We stepped out of the stall and Boots became frantic! She whinnied and ran around in circles! Bill had to go back in before she hurt her foal.

He was a vigorous colt and by this time he was trying to stand. Bill said, "Let's see if we can get him up and nursing. Maybe then she'll understand which one of us is hers."

While Bill kept Boots occupied—an easy task as all he had to do was stand there and let her adore him—the night watchman and I helped her colt up. It took us several attempts but on the fourth or fifth try he stayed up. We left him alone for a few minutes while he gathered up his coordination.

In the meantime, Boots was trying to push Bill toward her rump. She had evidently decided it was time for him to nurse.

Okay, we figured, she wants to nurse a foal. We'll give her one. I guided the colt back along her side and tried to aim his head in the general direction of a nipple. He was making sucking motions with his mouth, so he was ready. But as soon as he touched her, she *fired!* She kicked so hard that she cracked a board—an oak plank—in the wall of the stall. She didn't want this alien nursing her. Her "foal" was right there by her head, standing there on his own two legs.

"Let me do that," Bill said to me. The night man took the mare's head and Bill took over the guidance of the foal. She liked this. With Bill back there, she allowed the foal to be maneuvered until at last he had a nipple and nursed. After making sure he was going to stay attached, Bill stepped away from him toward Bootsie's head.

She either saw or smelled him there and realized if he was there then it couldn't be him back there nursing. She jerked away from the foal's grasp of her nipple and kicked again. Fortunately, the colt had lost his balance and fallen down when she jerked away, otherwise she probably would have injured him badly, or worse.

We tried it a couple more times and as long as she thought it was Bill who was nursing she was fine. Now Bootsie was not a silly young mare. This was her fifth or sixth foal and she'd never had a problem accepting any of them. She had been a good, protective mother—an excellent mother—each time. She had never wanted Bill—or any other person—to be "hers," but then no one else had ever smelled like a newborn foal.

We—or Bill—couldn't leave the stall. We couldn't leave her foal alone with her. We took the foal from the stall—she didn't bat an eye—and I tranquilized her. I told Bill to go to the house and shower well and change everything he had on, from cap to shoes.

Even though she was wobbly from the tranquilization and couldn't hold her head up, she nickered and whinnied when Bill left the stall but the chemicals kept her from getting too worked up. Meanwhile, her real foal wasn't very happy. From the next stall, he squealed and bounced around.

Bill returned in about thirty minutes, squeaky clean. He had used his daughter's scented soap and splashed on an abundance of high-powered cologne. Indeed, he smelled not unlike a flower shop and nothing like a horse of any age.

With him, he brought a plastic trash bag. "It's the shirt I had on," he explained. He went in the stall with the foal and rubbed the soiled clothing over the colt's back. The night man led the still-wobbly mare over to the foal's stall. The colt was glad to see her but she was noncommittal. Bill assisted the colt to a faucet so he could nurse and as the night man held the mare firmly, ready to react should she try to injure the baby, Bill backed away.

Boots was waking up a little now. Bill came over to where I was standing, easily within Bootsie's fields of vision and smell. She looked toward us but made no sound or no attempt to kick. After perhaps thirty seconds, the foal stopped nursing, walked to the other end of the stall, and lay down. Boots moved toward him and the night man allowed her to walk over, but he was still prepared to stop her from doing anything we didn't want. She sniffed her foal and nuzzled him and then she, too, lay down. The foal was more than two hours old now and this was the first time that Boots had attempted to go down since she delivered him.

She lay there and rocked back and forth a few times, then became very still for several minutes. Then, the colt teetered back to his feet and came over to her. She got up, shook the bedding off, and stood quietly as he nursed again. Bill was evidently weaned.

The colt grew well, sold well, and trained well, but Bill turned out to be sounder and probably just as fast.

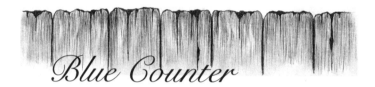

Blue Counter

BOYD CARPENTER WAS A *good* horse trainer. He got the absolute most out of a horse that could be gotten. If a horse had been an honest $5,000 claimer under another trainer, Boyd could usually get him to win for $6,500. He could turn high-priced claimers into allowance horses and allowance horses into stakes horses, but he rarely had the opportunity because very few owners gave him that kind of horse. If I had owned a racehorse while Boyd was alive, he would have been my trainer.

Boyd was just not "fashionable." Owners with money and good horses didn't want him to train for them. His typical owners operated on a shoestring and had only fair or worse horses. It didn't matter that an owner would send him a horse that was having trouble at $3,500 and a month later Boyd would have him holding his own at $5,000. I often wondered what he could have done with a really top horse.

One of Boyd's problems was his appearance. "Clothes make the man," I'm told, but Boyd wore old jeans well beyond the point that even I would wear them and I'm a slob. He wore old, holey T-shirts and floppy canvas shoes with holes in them where his toes rubbed.

And Boyd was old and stooped and walked with a two-legged limp. Very few people know this story because he didn't want anyone to know it, but Mary, his lady-friend/assistant trainer/groom/hot walker/pony girl/live-in companion, told it to me and had me promise not to let Boyd know I knew.

On a South Pacific Island in World War II, Boyd and several other soldiers were ambushed. Many were killed and those who weren't ran; they didn't check to see if anyone who had been shot was still alive, and even though Boyd called to them, they left him.

Boyd had only been hit in the legs—the knees—and he was left there. He was unable to walk, but he pulled himself along the ground on his elbows more than a mile back to where the camp was. Before he began his crawl, he checked his fallen companions. All were dead.

Boyd did walk again, albeit slowly and with great pain and difficulty. He had been a jockey before being drafted, but he knew that was not in his future, even before the crippling injuries, because he was not jockey-size. He was about five feet nine inches and could hold his weight below 120 as a young man, but it was difficult later on. He was racetrack-oriented and did not live in an area where steeplechasing took place. Also, he ballooned to about 160 pounds.

He loved horses and wanted to continue to work with them, so he became a blacksmith. That is *hard* work and not a job many sound men can handle, but Boyd was a good blacksmith. In knowing him, I suspect he would have been good at anything he chose to do.

Somewhere along the line—in the 1950s—he met Mary, who had just left her husband, a trainer himself. From what Mary told me, I don't think she ever divorced her husband. I know she and Boyd never married.

When they took up with each other, she saw how hard he worked as a farrier and how difficult it was for him. She suggested he become a trainer, but he told her he wouldn't be able to get any horses and he sure couldn't afford to buy any.

"Would you become a trainer if you could get some horses?" she asked.

He said he would. Mary knew that one of her estranged husband's owners was unhappy with the way his horses were performing, so she asked him to let

Boyd train them. A cheaper day rate was offered and with cheap horses—and these were real cheap—that's all-important.

So now Boyd had four horses to train. He got his trainer's license and did a good job for this man. These were $1,250 to $1,500 claimers, and they hadn't been winning, but Boyd got three of them to the winner's circle, one all the way up to $2,500.

Eventually, Boyd and Mary got more horses but never any of much quality and never enough in numbers. Once he had as many as fifteen head, but usually it was more like six or eight. Once or twice over the years, someone sent him a decent horse, but usually they were horses other trainers had not succeeded with. And most of the time, once Boyd had moved a horse up in class, the owner would then give the horse to another trainer, under whose care it would invariably drop back to where it had been before Boyd trained it.

His one chance at a good horse came some time in the mid-1960s, long before I was a vet. The horse was a two-year-old named Lin and Boyd trained him for his first five races. He won the first two, ran third, then won the next two, the last one a small stakes. At that point, Lin's owner gave him to a prominent, nationally known trainer at *twice* the rate Boyd was charging.

Lin went on to win another stakes race and one or two other races but wasn't the same horse at three and ended up running for about $15,000. Mary insisted he would have been a Derby contender if he had been left in Boyd's hands, but that's something no one will ever know.

I guess Boyd and Mary were in their late fifties when I began doing their vet work. It was in the 1970s and Boyd had about six horses, all very cheap claimers. They weren't doing well financially because horses that cheap don't earn much even when they win.

Once Mary asked me if I would neuter a kitten she had just gotten, so I went to their apartment. It was two rooms in the worst part of town, and it was so bad I was embarrassed. What's worse, it was obvious they were, too.

I had been doing their work for two or three years when I was asked to recommend a trainer. The man's name was Will Easton, and he owned a hardware store I dealt with. I got to know him very well because I am *not* a handy person and every time I needed to do something around the house I had to ask him what I needed and how to do it. (And I still usually botched the job.)

Will had spoken often of racing a horse or two and finally decided he would. He was fairly knowledgeable about the business end of racing and wanted to get in with a modest investment. He decided to find a trainer and have him claim a horse for him for about $5,000.

When he asked me, I told him to see Boyd. He did; they talked everything over, and Boyd claimed a horse named Rowdy Rag for him for $5,000.

Rowdy and Boyd won two races for Will and then he was claimed for $6,500. Will told Boyd to claim another one for him, and he took Missy L. for another $5,000. She, too, won two races and was taken for $5,000.

Will was happy. He was having fun and making money, although not much. This time he asked Boyd to step up the price a bit, so Boyd claimed Southland Duke for $7,500. Duke lasted a while—nearly a year—and won all the way up to $12,500 before he injured an ankle. After a layoff to heal, he was entered for $10,000, ran third, and was claimed.

Okay, Will was hooked on racing now. "Claim two," he directed Boyd, and he did. He took Mr. Earnest for $6,500 and Blue Counter for $10,000.

Mr. Earnest was a big disappointment. He couldn't win for $6,500 and was dropped to $5,000, then to $3,500, where he finally won and was claimed. It was the only horse Will had owned to that point on which he lost money.

But Blue Counter was another story. First of all, he was a delight. He wanted to play: He chewed on the shank when he was being led, he pushed people with his head to get their attention, he bounced when he went to the track simply because he felt so good.

When Boyd first brought him into his stable, he told me, "I think this can be an allowance horse." That appeared to be stretching it; Blue Counter was a six-year-old gelding that had run for as much as $17,500 a few years before but had seemed to settle in at around $10,000 for the last two years. He had been under three different trainers and that was where he seemed to belong: $10,000, plus or minus. "I've watched him for some time now," Boyd went on, "but I never had the money to claim him. And neither did any of my clients."

It would be a month at least before Boyd would run him because he needed to undo what previous trainers had done and institute his own training regimen. One day about three weeks after he claimed him, an exercise rider came to the training center from the racetrack near Cincinnati, where Blue had run. He saw the horse and told Boyd, "I don't know what's the truth, Mr. Carpenter, but I've heard things. Maybe you better x-ray his knees."

Okay, now we need a little anatomy lesson. The "knee" of a horse is the joint halfway down the front leg, but it's actually the carpus—our wrist. The joint in a horse analogous to the human knee is the stifle joint, located high on the hind leg. A lot of people think it's funny to call the wrist the knee and the knee the stifle, but that's the way it is in all mammals except us primates, so maybe it's actually funny that we call their knee our wrist, and so on. I guess it's all due to perspective.

Anyhow, Boyd asked me to look at Blue's knees. They looked and felt fine to me, but my borderline competence at lamenesses and joint problems is one of the reasons I left track work. "Let's x-ray them," he said, so we did.

Holy cow, what a mess! The left knee contained one fractured bone and an uncountable number of small chips. The right knee contained a spur and three or four chips.

"Is he ever lame?" I asked.

"No. He's never even taken a bad step that I've seen," Boyd replied.

"Does his regular exercise boy ever comment on how he feels under him?" Often a rider can feel a problem that's not apparent to an observer on the ground.

"He's never said nothin'," Boyd said. Just then the young man who exercised Boyd's horses rode by on another trainer's horse. "Hey, Jody," Boyd called, and the kid rode over. He asked him about Blue Counter and Jody said he "don't never take a bad step and feels great."

Boyd and I talked it over with Will, and the decision was made to go on and train the horse. About six weeks after he claimed him, Boyd put him in for $12,500. He finished second and ran sound. Two weeks later Boyd raised him to $15,000 and he won going away—by twelve lengths. And was sound.

A month later he ran Blue for $22,500 and he ran third, beaten only a length for it all. And again was sound. He brought him back in an allowance race a few weeks later and he won. By five.

Shortly after that race, Boyd asked me to step into his tack room. "Doc Kendall," he said, "there's a little stake comin' up next month and I wanna enter Blue. Do you think he'll hold up?"

I suggested we take another set of X rays and compare them with the first set to see if there were any further changes.

They were identical! Each chip was exactly where it had been, and the fractured pieces of carpal bone had not moved. I showed the films to a friend, a vet who does only leg work, and he explained it this way: The chips, which appeared to be floating in the joint fluid, were probably attached to the joint capsule, the tissue surrounding the entire joint. Floating chips are a problem, but attached chips aren't. The fracture must have healed, he said. He had seen several old fractures that were still evident on X rays but had, nonetheless, healed years before. And the spur was on a nonarticular surface and would never bother him.

"But he must've been one lame cookie at some point," he added.

So Boyd ran Blue in the stakes race and he won—by a head at eighteen to one. Will was ecstatic, but Boyd was more so, or so I thought. A few days later he came to me and asked, "You think Mr. Easton's gonna take Blue now that he's a stakes horse?" His lips were smiling but his eyes were worried.

I didn't know. I sure hoped not.

And he didn't. Will kept Blue with Boyd for four years. The old horse won one or two stakes a year through the age of eight, then dropped back to allowances at nine. In those four years he earned nearly a quarter-million dollars (in his first four years of racing he had won slightly less than $50,000), and Will's racing stable grew to five horses, all trained by Boyd. None were as good as Blue, but Will made money every year, and so did Boyd.

Blue's success and Will's other horses enabled Boyd and Mary to buy a small farm where they could live and take their tired and burned-out horses to be refreshed. They were a long way from rich, but for the first time in their lives, they owned a home.

By this time I had long since given up track work, although I still dropped by the training center occasionally to see Boyd and Mary and one or two others. By doing this, I was able to keep up with Blue's racing career. With the purchase of their farm, they asked if I would take care of their vet needs there. I was delighted to do it.

As the old horse was nearing ten, he was having trouble competing in allowance company. Still, each time he was sent to the track he would buck a little. It wasn't an attempt to unseat the rider, it was just the sheer pleasure he received from being ridden and exercised. No one concerned wanted to run him in a claiming race again, so Will retired him and gave him to Boyd and Mary, and they took him home. He lived a happy life on their small farm until he died at the age of eighteen. He had never been lame a single day.

Will eventually suffered a heart attack and was forced to get rid of his horses, and that was too bad because when he left racing that left Boyd and Mary back almost to where they were before he came along—"almost" because they had a home and they didn't before.

Mary passed away one winter day in late 1990, and I thought Boyd would follow shortly. He fell to pieces but eventually rallied. Every time I saw him, though, he told me how much he missed her. He was down to only three horses, and although I'm sure he was getting all there was to get out of them, they were doing very poorly. And so was he.

His knees—or should I say stifles?—became much worse as he got older. He had three operations through the VA, and after each one he was a little less able to get around. It was looking as if he would have to give up training—after all, he was approaching eighty and crippled—but his time ran out first. The fellow who had helped him since Mary's death found him sitting in his pickup truck in his driveway one morning in May 1995. He was dead.

Very few people went to his funeral: I was there, and his helper and an exercise rider and a couple of trainers. And Will came.

Boyd had no known relatives and none were found, so through whatever legal process was necessary, his farm was auctioned off. I remember reading the notice in the newspaper: "Absolute Auction. Blue Counter Farm."

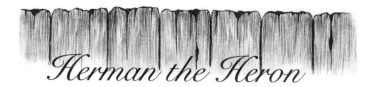

Herman the Heron

I LIKE BIRDS. I enjoy watching them, although I don't think I have the temperament or even the interest to be a bird-watcher, per se. It would drive me crazy to sit for hours waiting and hoping for a glimpse of a speckle-banded double-crested chirtle flitter, but if one happened to light on the branch of a nearby tree, I'd enjoy looking at it, even though I'd have no idea what it was.

And although I like sparrows and chickadees and other small species, I especially enjoy large birds: buzzards, swans, hawks, pelicans, etc. Owls are my favorites; one entire wall in our house is devoted to pictures—photos, prints, drawings—of owls. I think they're fascinating.

Early one morning—5:30 or so—I left the house on the way to my first call. At the end of our road there's a large, old, half-dead oak tree. By half-dead, I mean just that: Half the tree stands tall and majestic with long, luxuriant branches that are full of leaves in the spring and summer; the other half has nothing except a big hole in the trunk where a huge limb had once been.

The sun was still trying to rise as I drove near this tree on this particular morning. About ten feet from the tree, my headlights came upon something small flopping about in the road.

I stopped to see what it was. I do this because often these things are birds or small animals that have been hit by cars and are suffering. Unfortunately, they are rarely able to be saved, but at least I can end their pain. I don't like doing it, but I like less the thought of the unfortunate creatures lying there to be run over again or dying a slow death.

This one, though, was not injured. It was a baby owl trying his darnedest to fly and singularly not succeeding. From the tree came a loud and repetitious warning. I looked up, and in the hole in the trunk where the branch had once been was Momma Owl, obviously telling me to get away from her child.

Well, I couldn't leave him there in the road to be squished by a passing car. But although he was small, he still had that beak and those little talons, and I knew he would shred my hand if I tried to pick him up.

I found a broken branch in the tall grass on the side of the road. It was about twenty inches long, so I held it at one end and attempted to get the owlet to get on the other end. It was easy; the little guy took the proffered stick as a threat, and he attacked it with beak and talon. As he held on, squawking and biting, I lifted him out of the street and placed him and the stick in the hole in the tree, which was only about seven feet above the ground.

Mom, of course, took all my good intentions as the most evil sort of threat. She swooped at my head and shoulders several times but luckily for me caused no damage, other than to knock off my brand-new Detroit Tigers cap.

I don't know what became of the owlet and his family after that. I assume—and hope—that his next attempt at flight was more successful and that he went on to live a long and glorious life.

I'm going to change the subject now for a little while, but we'll get back to birds soon.

There are many magnificent horse farms here in central Kentucky, but one of the most beautiful was Belle Monde Farm. It was easily the prettiest one I ever worked for. It consisted of two parcels of land located about two miles apart.

Farm One consisted of about three hundred acres and was home to the young horses—the foals after weaning, the yearlings, and the two-year-olds in training until they left for the racetrack. Also on Farm One were the office, the manager's residence, and the owner's residence (more on him in a moment).

Farm Two was nearly six hundred acres and was where the broodmares lived, along with a few farm employees. There were four small houses there, and they were provided for the barn foremen and their families.

Also on Farm Two were two large and beautiful ponds. One, a pond of about an acre, was only a short distance behind the row of houses. The other was much smaller and was on the back of the farm where no horses were kept and people rarely went other than to periodically mow the vacant fields.

Belle Monde was owned by a Frenchman named Dr. Herman Goldfine. (I know; it doesn't sound French to me, either.) I never knew what kind of doctor Dr. Goldfine was, but he must have earned a good living from whatever it was he doctored because he had very expensive, high-quality mares and bred them to the best stallions.

Dr. Goldfine lived in France and only came to Kentucky about twice a year. At these times, he would insist on a lengthy meeting with the farm manager (Eric Bonetti) and the farm vet (me). Eric, who ruled the farm with an iron hand fifty weeks out of the year and appeared to a casual observer to be the owner, became a quivering jellyfish on these occasions. (I sometimes think there's an emotional test given to potential farm managers. If the results show that the candidate is stable and secure, he is blacklisted from ever becoming a farm manager.)

And to be honest, I didn't care for these meetings, either. For one thing, Dr. Goldfine could only speak conversational and business English, but not veterinary English, and he wanted to know *everything* about his horses. Eric's French was horrible and mine was only slightly better. I wouldn't starve if I found myself marooned in France (as long as the snails held out: *"Garcon, escargots, s'il vous plait."*) and I could tell everyone that my pen was on the table, although I don't believe I've ever needed that particular phrase in any language. Additionally, because in high school French all the boys had recently reached puberty, we learned (self-taught) to say, *"Voulez-vous couchez avec moi, Mademoiselle?"* I don't know how effective this question may have been, having never had the opportunity to converse with a French-speaking woman (and anyhow, I'd have been way too shy to say it), and somehow it never seemed appropriate when discussing equine health problems with Dr. Goldfine.

These meetings must have been frustrating for Dr. Goldfine, too. He wanted to know things such as why the mare he had just paid $300,000 for was not in foal or why the beautiful chestnut yearling was limping, and neither Eric nor I could explain these things satisfactorily in French. (We took notes at the meetings and several times I was tempted to leave my pen when I left just so I could go back later and tell him where it was, but I never did.)

Two of the barn foremen were actually forepersons: Eddie (real name, unfortunately: Edwina) and Belinda. They were in charge of the two twenty-four-stall broodmare barns and spent all their time on Farm Two. Eddie's husband was the farm's mechanic and Belinda's was in charge of breaking the yearlings. These two young women did excellent work, but our interest in them in these pages has nothing to do with their horse care.

Now back to birds. On the big pond behind the houses on Farm Two lived a heron. Or at least, I guessed it was a heron—Eddie said it was. He—Eddie also said it was a "he"—was a tall, grey, long-legged, majestic wading bird and he returned every summer for six or seven years. Eddie, who knew more about birds than anyone else on the farm, told us it was always the same bird that returned, anyhow, and I believe her.

The distance from the houses to the pond edge was only about fifty yards, and for the first few years of the heron's residency there, he would fly away whenever someone would come out of a back door. Eventually, it was discovered that he flew only as far as the smaller pond on the back of the farm.

After about three years, the heron earned a name: Herman, in honor of the farm's owner. Also, as the years passed, he became less quick to desert the big pond on the appearance of people. Instead of immediate, quick flight, it became a delayed, leisurely departure. Eventually, Herman wouldn't leave at all as long as the people didn't get too close or too loud. If they came down to the pond's edge, only then would he leave—slowly.

I had only seen Herman from the broodmare barns, a distance of maybe a hundred yards, and I wasn't sure I fully believed the stories Eddie and Belinda told me about his seeming "domestication." One day when Belinda was telling me she had gotten to within twelve to fifteen feet of Herman, I scoffed. "A wild heron isn't gonna let a person get that close," I said.

"When we finish here, I'll show you," she said.

After the horse work was done, I went to her house with her and then out the back door. "Now don't make a lot of noise," she cautioned. "Just walk quietly and act normal."

We walked down the slope toward the pond. Herman was standing about a foot deep in the water about ten or twelve feet offshore. He didn't seem to be watching us, but as we approached he became very still. We got to within ten feet of the waterline before he slowly rose out of the water and glided off toward the rear of the farm. I became a believer.

On slow days I'd go with Belinda or Eddie and watch Herman. As long as we didn't get too close—the limit seemed to be fifteen to twenty feet—he would just stand there motionless. Closer, and he would leave. If we remained fifty or so feet away, he carried on his normal activities; on two occasions we saw him catch a frog or a fish.

It came time once again for a Dr. Goldfine visit. I arrived at the main house for the scheduled meeting and found, in addition to Eric and the doctor, a third man, whom I knew slightly. His name was Robert Edelman, he was about sixty, British, and a bloodstock agent. He had married a local woman, a widow whose late husband had left her a horse farm and a lot of money.

And I learned that day, Robert Edelman was fairly fluent in French.

A lot of the conversation in that meeting was between Edelman and Dr. Goldfine in French. Edelman would ask a question of Eric or of me, we would answer, and he would translate for Dr. Goldfine. I don't know what was said (I heard no mention of snails, pens, or mademoiselles), but Dr. Goldfine frowned a lot and shook his head occasionally.

The next day Eric was fired. The day after that I was summoned to the farm office by Edelman and introduced to the new farm manager, one Billy Foley. I knew my tenure as Belle Monde's vet was over.

You see, Billy and I knew each other. Several years before, Billy attempted to train a few horses and I did some vet work for him. I was unimpressed with his horsemanship, and things came to a head one day when he sent a groom to get me. I went over to his training area and found him forcing a filly to walk.

She was "tied-up," a muscle condition resulting from overexertion. (This is a very simplified explanation.) A "tied-up" horse should *not* be walked; rather, it should be left where it is until it can be treated.

Perhaps if I had quietly taken Billy aside and explained that what he was doing was wrong I would still be Belle Monde's vet, but I didn't. When I saw the pain and distress the poor filly was experiencing, what I said, in front of the groom and within hearing of another trainer, was, "Damn, Billy! She's tied-up! Everyone knows you don't walk a tied-up horse!"

In other words, I embarrassed him in front of both an employee and a peer. He never asked me to do any vet work for him again.

As I said, when I saw Billy I knew I was out at Belle Monde. And I was. What I didn't know was why a horseman of borderline ability and knowledge (Billy) was replacing one of proven, if somewhat flamboyant, ability (Eric).

The reason was told to me a few weeks later by Eddie, who at the time she told me had also become an ex–Belle Monde employee. I bumped into her in the grocery store one day. It seems, she told me, that Billy was Edelman's stepson-in-law (he had married Edelman's wife's daughter).

Eddie also told me why she was no longer working there. And Belinda. And their husbands.

The story: The day after I was told my services were no longer needed, Billy toured the entire farm—both tracts. When he got to Farm Two, he saw Herman (the heron, not the owner). Eddie, who was his tour guide, proudly showed him how close they could get to the big heron.

"Man, that's great!" Billy reportedly said. "I'm gonna shoot him!" And he drove back to Farm One to get whatever type of gun he had.

Eddie said she didn't believe he really meant it, but she scared Herman off anyway. Within fifteen minutes Billy was back, shotgun in tow.

"Where's that bird?" he asked.

"He flew away," Eddie told him.

"He'll be back," Billy said. "They have their territory. I'll get him one of these days."

Apparently a conversation ensued, which developed into an argument and culminated in Eddie's resignation. Belinda had come upon them as they were nearly screaming at each other, and when she learned what they were arguing about, she joined Eddie's side. She also ended up resigning.

Billy countered in a mature manner: He fired their husbands on the spot. Fortunately, both men were quite accomplished at the things they did and found other employment within two weeks, as did Belinda. Eddie, who was pregnant, decided to remain unemployed until after the baby was born.

It took a few days for the two families to make their departures from Belle Monde, Eddie said, and during that time the two women went to the pond several times and scared Herman away. They even drove to the back of the farm to scare him off the pond there. Unfortunately, he was still hanging around when they finally had to leave.

"Why did he want to kill Herman?" I asked.

Eddie shook her head. She was almost in tears. "He said that's what birds are for," she answered.

I don't know if Billy killed Herman. I hope he didn't; I hope he shot himself in the foot instead.

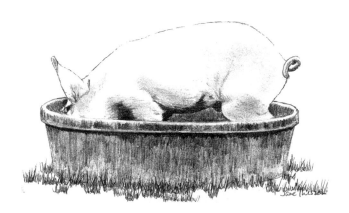

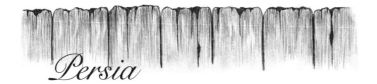

Persia

I DON'T KNOW THE STATISTICS, but the divorce rate is high among equine vets. I don't know how it compares with other fields of endeavor—I don't even know how it compares with other types of vets—but I think very few other lines of work produce as high a percentage of broken marriages.

The reasons are several and I'm sure I don't know them all, but here are some. Guys who do only track work are away from home a lot because very few areas have year-round racing. Those of us who do mostly reproductive work work fourteen to eighteen hours a day for four to five months of the year, then are constantly underfoot the rest of the time. Calls for all of us come at all hours of the day and night, so plans are hard to make and harder to keep. Meals are often missed. Kids' events are missed. Social engagements are missed. Sometimes even vacations are missed.

Another problem—a *big* problem—is fidelity. There are a lot of temptations out there. Horses attract women. Women of all ages. And over the years, I've observed that a higher percentage of women who are involved with horses is attractive. I have no idea why this is, but it's true.

And many times, the vet and the woman client are the only people present when treating a horse.

When I was younger and single and, in retrospect, more immature, when I was one-on-one with an attractive member of the opposite sex, some sort of pass was in order. Face it, I was a dirty ol' man well before my time. With age came mellowing, and I came to realize that perhaps there were other means of communicating with women.

Some in my profession never learn that, I guess, but in defense of my gender I think the problem, at least as it pertains to male horse doctors, lies as much with the female clients as it does with the vets.

Many times through the years, a woman client has openly flirted with me. A couple have even openly offered their services. One woman was so overt in her actions that I made it a point to have someone with me, usually one of the kids, whenever I knew I was going to her place.

For a while, I cared for the horses of a really pretty woman of about thirty. She was married and had a child and four horses. She hired a girl to help her with the farmwork, and the girl happened to be a friend of Laurie's.

This woman was very friendly and frequently asked me to come to her house for a snack or soft drink after the vet call was completed. When we talked, she stood close. She touched a lot—my arms, my hands, my shoulders, my legs occasionally. In time, I began to decline the invitations to the house. It seemed to be asking for it.

One day Laurie asked how I was getting along with this client. She was smiling a very mischievous smile as she asked it.

"Fine, I guess," I answered. "Why?"

"Jeannie told me something last night." Jeannie was Laurie's friend who worked for the woman.

It seems this woman and a friend, another very attractive woman whom I had met at my client's farm two or three times, were having a contest to see which one could seduce her vet first.

I don't know who the other gal's vet was, nor do I know if she seduced him. I do know, if she didn't, the contest was a tie.

⌀∞∘

One day I received a call from Dr. Peter Baldwin, who had been one of my teachers in vet school years before. He was one of the equine clinicians.

"Grant," he began, "you can thank me later."

"For what?" I asked.

"I'm sending you a client. She's moving to your area."

He told me about her. Her husband was a physician and had been hired by the University of Kentucky hospital. She had one horse, an Arabian mare, which she dearly loved and took great care of.

A one-horse client wasn't anything to get excited about and I wondered why Pete had even called to tell me, but I thanked him.

"Don't thank me yet," he said. "Wait'll you see her." He chuckled. I thought he meant the mare.

Maybe two weeks later, I got a call from a woman. She said her name was Sandy Pitts and she was new to Lexington and needed a vet. I had nearly forgotten about Pete's call and had forgotten the name he told me, but then she said, "Dr. Baldwin recommended you."

Well, to say the least, my curiosity was piqued. I still thought Pete had meant the mare, but I found out otherwise. She asked if I could come and check her mare, named Persia, and see if she had made the trip in good shape. I told her I'd be there the next morning.

Sandy Pitts was, in a word, a knockout, possibly one of the two or three most beautiful women I've ever seen. Right away I knew that Pete had not been talking about the mare. My wife will read this one of these days and she's very, very pretty, and I hope she understands. Sandy was just another level. She's the only woman that Tommy Williams, who still rode with me occasionally in those days, ever commented on.

The Pitts family had not found a place to buy yet, so Sandy kept Persia at a farm where several others kept their pleasure horses. I checked the mare and she had made the six-hundred-mile trailer ride in fine shape.

Persia was a very handsome mare, but I know little about Arabians, so I have no idea how good a specimen she was. She was a lovely dappled grey (a lot of Arabians are grey, I've noticed) and a little larger than most of the members of her breed I've worked on. And she had a good, gentle disposition, in contrast to the easily spooked, flighty Arabians I had encountered before.

Sandy told me what vaccinations Persia had received and when she had been wormed and asked me to make her a schedule. I did.

Two weeks later I wormed her (Persia, not Sandy). It was a slow day and no one else was at the barn, so I hung around and Sandy and I talked for maybe a half hour. I enjoy the company of pretty women. I have never seen anything wrong with that.

A few days later, Sandy called and said Persia was acting "funny." Thinking it might be colic, I got there as soon as I could, only to find a seemingly normal mare. "She's acting fine now," Sandy explained. "She straightened up just a few minutes ago."

An examination showed that she was, indeed, fine. And I stayed and talked for about fifteen minutes.

In another two or three days, Persia was acting "funny" again, and again she was okay when I got there.

The mysterious ailment flared up about twice a week for several weeks. One day, when once again Persia was in good health when I got there, Sandy asked if I'd like something to drink. It was a hot day and I said, "Yeah. A Coke would go good right now."

"No, silly," she said. "I mean a real drink." She pulled out a thermos bottle.

"What's that?"

"Manhattans."

I'm not a drinker. I used to have the occasional screwdriver, but the vodka just ruined a perfectly good glass of orange juice. And I'm a cheap drunk. Wave a cork under my nose and I'm ready to go curl up in a corner and sleep it off. So I quit drinking screwdrivers.

And other than a town in Kansas and some part of New York City, I didn't know what a Manhattan was, but I took one. (She had conveniently brought along two plastic cups.)

Boy, was it terrible! I tried to sip it politely and not make faces, but it was tough. Sandy, meanwhile, drank hers down without so much as a wince.

"You know something I've wondered?" she asked, smiling very sweetly and moving close to me.

I had no idea, so I said, "No."

"I wonder what it would be like if we kissed." She moved her body right on up to mine, to the point where I didn't have to look to know that she had certain very feminine contours.

Now to be perfectly honest, I had wondered the same thing. She was a beautiful woman and I was still alive. It would take a dead man not to think along those lines when confronted with Sandy.

Oh, boy, I thought, where's a kid when you need one?

But I was married and a good boy, so I backed away and escaped with my virtue intact. "That was a close one," I said to myself as I drove away. I was feeling pretty certain that Persia was not really having bouts of colic or whatever. I'm quick that way.

Sandy was persistent. Two days—nights—later she called again. It was nearly 9 P.M. and I was giving strong thought to going to bed.

"Persia's acting funny again," she said.

"I don't think so," I told her.

"Oh, she is! She's looking at her side and pacing! Something's wrong with her."

I didn't have a choice. I had to go. Miraculously, Persia was better when I got there. Sandy wanted to talk, but I told her I had to get home. We got in our cars and headed out the driveway and onto the road.

About a quarter mile from the farm, there was a road to the right. Why it was there I don't know because it didn't go anywhere. It was maybe a half-mile long and there weren't even any houses on it.

I was behind Sandy as we headed toward the main road back into town. As she reached the aforementioned side road, she slammed on her brakes and hopped out of her car. I got out to see what was going on.

"Did you see it!?" she said.

"Did I see what?"

"The dog! I think I hit a dog!"

"I didn't see any dog."

"Yes. It ran down the road! It may be hurt! We have to find it!"

Well, if there was a hurt dog I couldn't leave it, although I had no idea how we could possibly find it. It was after 10 P.M. by this time, and there was only a slice of moon, but still, I had to try.

We drove our cars slowly to the end of the side road. No dog. She got out of her car and walked back to mine. She had a flashlight and a blanket in her hands.

"I think he went over there," she said, pointing the flashlight into a stand of trees off to one side.

"What's the blanket for?" I asked.

"If he's hurt, we may have to wrap him up. Come on."

Some days I'm dumber than others. I followed her.

"Gosh, it's dark and eerie," she said, and leaned up against me as we walked. She was shining the flashlight ahead of us.

We were maybe fifty yards off the road and in the trees when we heard a car drive up. She shut off the light. My first thought was that my car with all my veterinary equipment was standing there unattended. I turned to go back to it.

"That's my husband!" Sandy gulped.

"Oh, good," I said. "Let's go."

"No!" she whispered and grabbed my arm to hold me back. "He'll kill us!"

It was at this point that it dawned on me that there probably was no injured dog. I doubted if her husband would actually kill us, but I had never met him, and for all I knew he was six-eight and weighed 250 pounds. Maybe he would maim us, though, so I stopped.

After ten minutes, during which time he walked around the cars and shone a flashlight off into the darkness, he drove off and Sandy breathed again.

"God, that was close!" she said. "Here. Take this." She handed me the blanket. "If he finds it in my car, I don't know what he'll do."

"Just leave it here," I suggested.

"No. If he comes back here in the daylight, he'll find it. And he'll know."

I started to ask what he would know, but I thought better of it. I was beginning to feel that theirs was not a marriage built on mutual trust.

When I got home it was after 11 P.M. My wife was waiting up.

"Do you know a Dr. Pitts?" she asked.

I told her I knew of him. It seems he called and asked her if she knew where I was. He described a car and asked if it was mine. (It was.) For some reason, she wanted to know what was going on.

I told her what had happened and she believed me. I hope. I even gave her the blanket.

Believe it or not, Sandy called again three days later. Persia was acting funny. I told her I didn't think so, but she insisted. I went. Persia was fine.

"That was close the other night," Sandy said. "What's the matter? Don't you think I'm attractive?"

I assured her that I thought she was *very* attractive. "But," I said, "we're both married and I love my wife. If I was single—and you were single—I would certainly be interested, but we're not and we can't." And I left.

Four days passed. That was the longest period in which Sandy hadn't called for weeks. I figured she finally got the message.

But the on the fifth day, right at dinnertime, she called. "Persia's acting funny," she said. "It's real this time."

"Oh, come on, Sandy." I wasn't going to bite again.

"No, Grant. It's real. She's down and rolling."

"Just watch her," I said, and hung up.

Twenty minutes later she called again. "Grant, you *have* to come! She won't get up."

"She'll be okay in a few minutes," I said, and hung up again.

I told my wife. "Maybe you'd better go," she said.

I sighed. "If she calls again, I guess I will."

She called back in another half hour. "She's really awful," she sobbed. Very convincing sobbing, too. "Please come."

I went. I kicked myself all the way there because I knew Persia would be fine.

But she wasn't. She was in a *bad* way. It turned out to be a twisted intestine, and we rushed her to surgery. We were able to save her, but it was touch-and-go for several days. Getting her on the table an hour earlier would definitely have made a big difference in ease of surgery, recovery time, and size of vet bill. It was my fault for not responding sooner, but it was Sandy's fault, too, for crying wolf all those times.

In fact, at first I thought Persia was going to die. I didn't sleep well until she was out of the woods. When it was apparent that she would recover, I told Sandy that she needed to find another vet.

Please don't think the above described incidents with women clients are typical. I have had many pretty women clients who either didn't try to seduce me even if they wanted to, or found the idea not to their liking. I prefer to think they were able to control their emotions.

And as I've gotten older, I find that it's not nearly as big a problem.

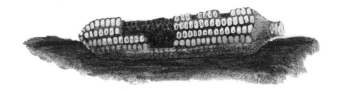

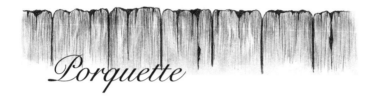

Porquette

THE FARM ACROSS THE ROAD from us had cattle roaming its fields for years. I tried not to notice, but they were always there and ruined an otherwise perfectly good rural neighborhood.

But one day several years ago I noticed that there were no cows within sight when I looked out across the road from our front window.

"Where are the cows?" I asked no one in particular.

"Geez, Dad!" my son said in an exasperated manner. "There haven't been any cows over there for days."

"More'n a week," added my daughter in a voice that sounded as if she wanted to add, "Dumb ol' Dad."

I don't know if I was so used to their being there that I hadn't paid attention, or if my aversion to the beasts caused me to unconsciously turn my head away when I passed there, but I honestly hadn't seen that they were gone before that moment.

They'd be back, though. I knew that. Maybe not the same cows, but it didn't matter. A cow is a cow. You see one cow, you've seen 'em all. But several more days passed and the field remained empty. The tension was building. I *knew* they'd be there, but when? The suspense mounted. I'd stand in our living room, looking out over our front pasture, across the road, and into the empty field . . . waiting. The cows would come.

Now, instead of averting my eyes as I drove past that field, I would look into it. Every morning I would look out the front window, just in case they had moved in some cows overnight. It became a fixation. One day my wife called me on my mobile phone to ask me to get a few things at the grocery store, and I heard myself ask, "Have they moved any cattle in across the street yet?"

And then one afternoon when I got home early, I looked out the window to the field across the road. There, behind the barn on the back of the property, I saw them: trucks. Two trucks. *Livestock* trucks. I hadn't seen them from the road as I drove by because of the lay of the land, but our house sits on a small rise and the view is considerably expanded.

Through the pall of gloom that I felt falling over me, I said to the empty room, "They're back."

I turned to other things. I knew depression would set in quickly if I continued to dwell on cows as neighbors, so I went to the barn to talk to the horses. That's usually a waste, though; as much as I like them, they're terrible conversationalists. They're not even very good listeners.

When I returned to the house a half hour later, the kids had gotten home from school.

"Hey, Dad," my son said, "did you see what they got across the street?"

Through the heavy curtain of woe and despair, my hollow voice sounded distant as I answered, "Yes. Isn't it awful?"

"Awful? Dad, you always said you *liked* pigs!" he exclaimed.

Pigs!? I rushed to the front window. Yes, it was pigs! Maybe a dozen pigs! Not cows!

I don't mean to insinuate that, given a choice, I would choose a pig farm for a neighbor, even though I do like pigs. I wouldn't. It might not even be in the Top Ten, but a pig farm versus a cattle farm is no contest.

As I said, I like pigs. They're intelligent, clean, and relatively easy to care for. Unfortunately, they're also big and smelly. You can't have everything.

To change the subject for a moment, our nearest neighbors, as far as the proximity of the house is concerned, are the Mannings—Roy and, believe it or not, Circe. They live on two acres right next to our property; in fact, the edge of our driveway actually overlaps the property line a few inches.

How they acquired two acres is a question that has never been answered. The laws (rules, statutes, or whatever) of our county state clearly that houses cannot be built on fewer than five acres. You can't even *sell* parcels smaller than five acres. So not only do I not know how the Mannings built on two acres, I don't even know how they bought it.

That's neither here nor there, however. The Mannings built a barn on their two acres with the intention of boarding pleasure horses. Two acres, of course, gives neither sufficient pasture space nor a place to ride, so the barn—a nice eight-stall barn—sat empty.

We're almost back to the pigs. Be patient.

When you build a fence—any kind of fence—for livestock—any kind of livestock—put the materials—planks, wire, whatever—*inside* the posts. Animals lean against the fences and they push. If the fence material is outside the posts, the nails or staples are loosened and the planks or wire come loose. And the animals may get out.

The fence across the road was of what I have always called hog wire, but I have come to learn that most people call it box wire. Properly built and maintained, it makes a great fence for any kind of livestock. This one, however, was neither properly built nor maintained. The wire was on the outside of the posts, which were old and rotting, and the nails were loose and rusted and the victims of years of being leaned on by cows.

Okay, now we're back to the pigs. All the pigs that moved in were pregnant sows and eventually they farrowed, and the dozen or so became maybe a hundred.

And they pushed against the fence, a fence built incorrectly and already weakened by years of cattle pushing against it.

One day Circe Manning came home from shopping and there was a piglet in the road, running (actually, limping) frantically up and down the fence line, squealing. This was a *little* pig—maybe three weeks old—so Circe picked it up and placed it in a box in her garage.

The owner of the pigs didn't live on the farm. Either he or an employee would come and tend to the animals each day, but usually no one was there. Circe called the owner's home, told him about finding the piglet outside the fence, and added, "It's limping."

The owner drove out to claim his pig, but when he saw it, he told Circe that it would be no good to him with a bad leg, so he'd just shoot it. Circe asked if she could have it instead of him killing it. "Sure," he said, "for ten dollars."

"But you're going to kill it and you won't get anything," she protested.

"It's my pig and I can do what I want to," he said. "Take it or leave it."

She gave him ten dollars.

I learned of this a few minutes later when Circe called me on my mobile phone and asked if I could come and look at her piglet and tell her how to care for it.

When I saw the little pig (a girl) walk, I saw she wasn't using her left hind leg much. I took an X ray and found a small fracture in the left side of the pelvis. A full-grown pig, or even an adolescent, would never be able to withstand an injury such as this—too much weight—but a baby this size would heal, I was sure. I told Circe to confine the piglet in a small area—a box would be good—so she wouldn't be able to move around much. (We didn't know the cause of the injury. Maybe her mother had lain on her or maybe a car had hit her when she got through the fence.)

Circe did as I suggested, and she and Roy bottle-fed the baby for a couple of weeks. By then, the limp had improved considerably and she was doing well on solid food. It was obvious she would be able to lead a fairly normal life.

So now the Mannings had a pet pig. And they had an empty eight-stall barn.

Roy built a fence around the barn so their pig, now named Porquette, could move from the garage. (Pigs outgrow garages very quickly.) He built it out of hog wire, which, as I said, makes a great fence. But he built it wrong. The wire was on the outside of the posts.

Porquette grew and thrived in her eight-stall barn and quarter-acre paddock. Roy and Circe were good pig owners. They fed her well and petted her and loved her and Porquette loved it.

My wife is big on not wasting anything. If it's recyclable, she recycles it. If it's compostable, she composts it. More people should be this way.

One day she told me to bring a bucket from the barn and she'd save our nonmeat leftovers for Porquette. (The meat leftovers went in the dogs' meals.) Every two or three days, one of the kids would take the bucket up to Porquette's paddock and dump it over the fence. She loved it and the Mannings appreciated it.

The bearer of the slop was usually our daughter, and although we didn't realize it at the time, she created a problem. She was too short to comfortably reach over the fence to dump the bucket, so she'd stand on tiptoes and pour the garbage *just* over the wire. It fell straight down, right to where the hog wire met the ground, and some would even bounce back through the fence to where Porquette couldn't reach it easily.

There is a reason people who eat a lot are called "pigs." Porquette liked her food. In her attempts to get all that was poured from the bucket, she would try to push the wire out of her way—the wire that was on the *wrong* side of the posts.

And she knew what the bucket meant: food!

I don't know how good pig vision is. Maybe we were told in school, but I don't think so. Porquette's must have been pretty good, though, because when

Laurie or I would feed the horses, Porquette, from nearly a hundred feet away, would start to squeal whenever we carried buckets. If no bucket was in sight, she was silent.

One afternoon when Laurie had to leave early for some reason, I was feeding. It was a beautiful day and I'm kind of lazy, so I saw no reason why the horses had to come in the barn to eat when it was so much easier to feed them outside.

Porquette saw me carrying the bucket, not once but several times, as I went from field to field. I guess it was too much for her. Squealing and pushing against the already weakened fence, where her slop had always been dumped, she suddenly found herself free! Free and in sight was the purveyor of gustatory delights: the bucket!

She zoomed to me, or I should say, to the bucket I was carrying. The Mannings weren't home, so I held the bucket just out of her reach and walked into our barn and into a stall.

She followed eagerly and I gave her a little of the sweet feed just before I closed her in. When Roy and Circe came home, I told them what had happened. Roy repaired the fence, and we led Porquette back home by holding the bucket just ahead of her.

Porquette had attained considerable size by this time—probably in excess of 200 pounds—and as we were leading her home, Roy said to me, "We've decided to breed Porquette."

Somehow that didn't seem like a good idea. I knew they wouldn't make sausage out of her offspring and her quarter-acre lot wasn't big enough to accommodate too many pigs. But at least each could have its own stall.

He went on. "We've arranged to have her artificially inseminated. A litter of pigs will be fun."

And they went ahead and did it. The AI man came and went and Porquette conceived. A sow's farrowing date is easily calculated. Gestation is 114 days, or three months, three weeks, and three days.

Beginning on day 110, though, Roy and Circe alternated spending the night with Porquette in the barn. Circe took 110, so she was on duty on the night of 114 when Porquette went into labor.

But nothing came. She went to the house and got Roy, who agreed with her that nothing was coming.

You know what happened next. They called me. It was after two in the morning in late August. The foaling season was over, and I hadn't expected a sleep interruption for another five to six months anyhow.

But I went right over. I expected to find the first pig stuck sideways—a real common problem with pigs. Once the first one is straightened, the rest pop right out.

But that's not what I found because I could barely get my hand in to find anything.

The birth canal was too narrow. *Way* too narrow. Evidently the pelvic fracture that had occurred when she was a baby had healed so that the space between the two sides of the pelvis—the birth canal—was much smaller than it should have been.

Using the lube I use to palpate mares, I was finally able to get my hand in far enough to find that the first piglet's presentation was normal. With much effort and much lube, and using only my fingertips, I was able to deliver the six babies she was carrying, but it was nearly a total tragedy.

Five of the piglets were injured so badly getting them through the compromised space that they died within minutes. And Porquette's vaginal wall was lacerated from trying to put things that were too large through a space that was too small. Infection set in quickly and that, combined with shock from the stress of the difficult farrowing, was too much for her. She died three days later.

Circe was hysterical that night and Roy close to it. They mourned Porquette's loss for days, but they couldn't dwell on it for long because they had another responsibility.

Porquette's sixth and final piglet was a runt, a little female. So little, in fact, that there *was* room for her to fit through the narrowed space.

Porquette lived long enough for her piglet to nurse and get the colostrum she needed and then the baby, like her mother, became bottle-fed.

They named her Porcina and she's done well. She has her own eight-stall barn and her own quarter-acre paddock, and she gets a bucket of leftover veggies two or three times a week. The fence has been fixed so that it's now escape-proof, but like Porquette before her, she knows what that bucket means.

And you'd never know that she was a runt. I guess she must weigh 300 pounds now. There has been no mention of breeding her.

The pigs eventually were removed from across the road. About a month later, the cows were back. I knew they'd be back.

The fence has never been repaired, and I live in fear that a calf will get out, somehow and Circe will find it.

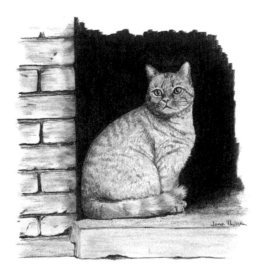

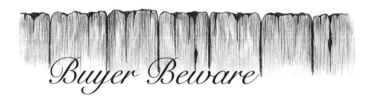

Buyer Beware

IN AN IDEAL WORLD, only top mares would be owned and bred. In an ideal world, everyone would have enough money to purchase a top mare. In an ideal world, I would still be a veterinarian, but first I would have been a Hall of Fame baseball player.

But it's not an ideal world. Cheap mares are owned and bred, most people can't afford a top mare, and my fastball wasn't.

Ignoring my baseball aspirations, there are a lot of nonwealthy people out there who want to breed Thoroughbreds and can't afford a six-figure mare, or even a five-figure mare. There's no reason why they shouldn't own a mare, or mares, though, if they're aware of what they're doing and the odds *against* anything more than moderate success, if that. Owning a mare, planning a mating, raising a foal—these are enjoyable, maybe even therapeutic in some cases.

The secret, I think, is to acquire the best-quality mare that can be justified with the money available to spend. If $15,000 is all that can be spent, buy accordingly. If $5,000 is the limit, buy the best $5,000 mare that can be found. If the person is unsure, there's advice out there: agents. A good, honest agent more than earns his (or her) commission.

All agents, however, are not good or honest.

Many years ago, a client of mine—Bart was his name—was an agent who also owned a farm. He had mares that he had purchased for his clients come and go, and I never knew anything about his dealings. He and his clients always paid on time, and that was good enough for me.

At the November breeding stock sales one year, he came to me with a new client. He introduced us and said, "Mr. Weldon intends to buy some mares and board them with me. He wanted to meet the vet who will care for them."

That was good news: a commission and boarders for him and mares to work on for me.

"I plan to spend $125,000, more or less," Weldon said.

"Great," I responded. "You should be able to get a pretty nice mare or two for that."

"Oh, no," he said. "Bart says I should buy about twenty."

I started to say something, but Bart hurried him off. "I'll have you check the mares after we've bought them," he called back over his shoulder. I was dumbfounded.

A half hour later, I ran into Bart, *sans* Weldon, in the rest room. He laughed. "Grant, you almost screwed up," he said. He explained what he was up to. He would receive the same commission from Weldon on his $125,000 whether it was spent on one mare or 125, but the board on twenty would be vastly greater than the board on one or two. And he added, I would also benefit more from twenty than from a couple; charging for worming, vaccinating, palpating, culturing, and all the other various and sundry health care procedures on twenty mares and their offspring could well put me in another tax bracket, he said. I told him I thought he was screwing the guy. "That's the horse business," he told me, and winked.

Bart purchased twenty-six mares for Weldon and spent $127,000 of the man's money. Occasionally, a carefully selected $5,000 mare can be a good buy, but two dozen randomly purchased cannot be. None of the twenty-six had been a decent racehorse, and none had ever produced anything that could run enough to justify training bills. If I was as good a person as I sometimes profess to be, I would have quit then and never worked on them, but I'm not and I didn't. I guess I rationalized that someone would do the vet work and charge for it; it might as well be me. And it was, even though I felt guilty about it each time I realized what the poor guy was having to spend. Mr. Weldon's vet bills would sometimes run as much as $5,000 a month during the breeding season.

Within four years Weldon was completely disillusioned, out of the horse business, and nearly broke. Fifteen dollars a day board per horse for twenty-six mares and their offspring, not to mention stud fees and those horrendous vet bills, can put a dent in anyone's bank account. The foals the mares produced were worth little; most of them sold for $1,000 to $3,000. When he sold out, the twenty-six mares that had averaged about $5,000 each when he bought them were older and still had not produced anything worth the expense as far as runners were concerned; they averaged just over $3,500 each.

It should have been a crime, but it was, as Bart said many times, "the horse business." I ended my association with him.

A few years later, a local man—Jon—decided he wanted to enter the horse business. He had made a lot of money in the business world and knew that he needed decent-quality mares to make a go of it, so he decided to buy five or six in the $50,000 to $70,000 range.

He was unfamiliar with conformation, pedigrees, and the vagaries of auctions, so he wisely consulted an agent, into whose hands he placed his entire equine financial operation: purchase of mares, acquisition of stallion seasons, and the promise to let the agent sell his yearlings for him when the time came.

Jon had his own farm—he had inherited it—but it was just open land that had been used for crops years ago and nothing had been on it for decades. He built proper barns and fences for his new undertaking. A few hundred thousand dollars were spent. I came into the picture when Jon asked an adjacent farm owner, my friend Fred Ballenger, to suggest a vet. I was Fred's vet, so he suggested me.

Later, Fred, while checking sale prices in one of the weekly Thoroughbred industry magazines, noticed that one of Jon's mares, for which Jon had said he paid $55,000, was recorded as RNA at $45,000. He looked up Jon's other mares; each one had been RNA at $10,000 *below* the price Jon claimed he had paid. (RNA is the notation the sales company makes in the sale summaries for a horse that did not bring the amount the seller wanted and, therefore, did not sell; it stands for "Reserve Not Attained.")

Not knowing what was going on—maybe Jon reported inflated prices out of ego—he didn't say anything to him about it. He mentioned it to me one day, but I didn't understand it, either.

The agent lined up some nice stallions for Jon, but I had the feeling, and Fred mentioned it, too, that maybe they were just a hair below the quality the mares warranted. Fortunately, all five mares conceived. However, the following spring, one delivered live twins on a contract that negated the fee (which had been paid September 1) if twins were not registered. Most stallion contracts stipulate "live foal guarantee," and many have the twin provision included.

Jon called his agent and requested a refund of the $15,000 stud fee. Many weeks passed. After several requests, the agent finally told him that the stud farm would not refund the fee and he was "working on it."

Jon decided to go to the source. He contacted the stud farm. They said they had heard nothing from the agent and knew nothing about the twins, but told him the refund would be made immediately on receiving a veterinary certificate attesting to the fact that live twins had been born to his mare. I gave him another certificate (the first one had been given to the agent), and a few days later Jon received a check for $7,500.

He was ticked. No, actually, he was irate. He called back and demanded his remaining $7,500. He was informed that the contract the agent had signed called for only a $7,500 fee, not the $15,000 the agent had charged Jon. He went to the stud farm in person and saw the contract with the agent's signature. The stud farm's general manager sympathized with him for having the twins and told Jon it hurt them, too, because the mare concerned was far better than what the stallion normally had bred to him. "This mare could easily be bred to a $25,000 stud," he said.

Subsequent inquiries at other farms revealed that the other four stallion contracts had been handled in the same manner: The agent had doubled the price in each case.

On hearing of this, Fred told Jon about the RNA prices he had seen. Jon contacted the sellers individually and learned that the agent had approached each of them after their mares went through the ring unsold and offered them $5,000 *more* than the RNA price, which they accepted. The agent then told Jon the price was actually $10,000 more than the RNA and pocketed the additional $5,000. He also charged Jon his 10 percent commission on the price he reported ($10,000 more than the RNA).

Legal action ensued and Jon recovered a portion of his money, but it took nearly three years and thousands of dollars in legal fees. He was so disenchanted that he, too, left the horse business. Fortunately, his mares kept their value and their foals were worth a little, too, so he actually came out in pretty good shape.

This is not an indictment of all agents. Good ones are invaluable, but a newcomer must be careful when choosing one, and he must authorize the agent to buy the best horses his wallet can afford—no more, no less. If he needs advice on matings and marketing, he should get it. After that, it's up to him to enjoy owning them. It's not an ideal world, but the right advice and the right horses can make it pretty doggoned good.

I couldn't hit a fastball, either.

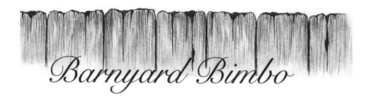

Barnyard Bimbo

THERE ARE MANY THINGS in this life that I don't understand, but revealing my ignorance is not the purpose of these epistles. I will go into one, however, and it has nothing to do with animals.

This particular thing that I have trouble with is really twofold: pronunciation and silent letters. They often go hand in hand.

Take, for instance, Hall of Fame outfielder Carl Yastrzemski. It's not pronounced as it's spelled because the z is silent. But if it's silent, why is it there?

Then there are names such as Dr. Rzegn's. Again, the z is silent (z, it seems, is often the culprit), but here the other letters aren't pronounced correctly, either. He says it's "Ring," but if I had to choose a pronunciation (and knowing to ignore the z), I'd have to say "Rain."

And how about Lech Walesa, the Polish statesman? Everyone pronounces it "WaleNsa." Why? There's no n there at all.

Bear with me and we'll eventually get to the story of the horse named Barnyard Bimbo (pronounced just as it's spelled). Her owner was a very nice guy named Bob (no pronunciation problem here, either) Schoenbourn. If that was my name, I think I'd pronounce it "Shoneborn," but he said it's pronounced "Shanebern." So why isn't it spelled "Shanebern"?

Okay, on with the story.

Bob owned a mare named Barnyard Bimbo. I never asked how she got that name; maybe I should have.

She came under my veterinary care a year after she had been retired as a racehorse when Bob moved her from the farm where she had been boarded to the farm of one of my clients, a good horseman named Sam Pavlecik ("Pavlichek"). She had not been bred that first year because, Bob was told by the other farm, "she never really came into a good heat."

Bimbo had been a very useful—and sound—race mare. She ran six years and earned just over $100,000 the hard way—roughly a dollar a start. Bob held no illusions about her class—she was a $20,000 to $30,000 claimer at her best—but he hoped she would reproduce her soundness. In six years, she made 115 starts and never took a bad step.

When she arrived at Sam's farm, he turned her out in a paddock with two other maidens, one of which happened to be in season. Bimbo went to her immediately, snorting and prancing like a stallion, and tried to mount her. This was met with a certain amount of disapproval from the in-season maiden, which had never been jumped before.

At great risk to himself, Sam removed the in-heat filly (he couldn't catch Bimbo), but then Bimbo attacked the other maiden in the field. Once he got that one out, too, Bimbo was catchable but she tried to bite him. She was given her own paddock.

I heard about this a couple of days later. It was February and the breeding season was just getting ready to start and some mares were coming in heat, so once again I actually had reason to get up in the mornings.

This particular day Sam had two mares in season: the previously mentioned maiden and a barren board mare that had just arrived from out of state. After culturing those two, Sam said, "Watch me tease that mare," pointing to a stall at the far end of the barn.

As soon as he led the teaser into the barn, a roar that sounded like a wild bull came from the end of the barn. Then there was a crash followed by another roar.

"Go look at her," Sam told me. He was standing there with the teaser some forty feet from the mare. I looked in at her. She had her ears back and her teeth bared and was attempting to rear, but the stall ceiling was too low; in between attempts, she kicked the walls.

He took the teaser back out, returned, and got this wild mare out, muzzling her. "Watch this," he said, and led her up the aisle to the mares we had just cultured.

She teased them as well as any stallion I had ever seen. When he finally got her back to her stall, not an easy task because she did not want to leave the mares, he asked, "What's wrong with her?"

I didn't know. He told me what he knew about her at that point.

She didn't improve. By late April she hadn't changed. She was perhaps slightly less aggressive toward people but still could not be turned out with other mares or approached by the teaser. A couple of times I tried to palpate her, but she reared and kicked so violently, even with tranquilization, that it was not possible. I told Sam that, maybe, with stocks I *might* try it again.

Sam called the farm that had boarded her the previous year. She had indeed not come into a "good heat" while there. Or any other kind. They had told Bob he had to move her because she had injured one of their employees and twice had broken stall doors when they tried to tease her. Their vet had tried to examine her a couple of times and had been unable to do it. Finally, he refused to try anymore.

I asked Sam to try to find out about her racing days. Had she always been aggressive? Had she suffered any illnesses or injuries? Had she been on any medications?

He talked with Bob. No, she had not always been aggressive, only since she was three (she was now nine). No, she had never been sick or injured. No, she had not been on any medications, "only vitamins and stuff to pick her head up."

"What kind of 'stuff'?" I asked.

Bob didn't know, but he had all his vet bills from her racing career. He dug them out and brought them to Sam's farm. The "stuff" was a commonly used long-acting injectable anabolic agent, commonly termed a *steroid*. It had been given to Barnyard Bimbo every three weeks from the age of three through the age of seven. Five years.

In the last few years, anabolic steroids have been making headlines. An Olympic athlete tested positive for them. A former pro football player's death was linked to their use in his younger days. (This may be coincidental or it may not: The average life expectancy of an NFL lineman is fifty-four years.) Some high school coaches have been charged with giving them to their players.

The evidence of anabolic abuse in humans is there. It (abuse) also exists in horses, but it's much more difficult to document. Barnyard Bimbo was definitely such a case. The problem, of course, is not the fault of the drug, no more than it is the fault of the needle and syringe used to deliver it.

Anabolics are exceptionally useful products when used for their intended purpose, namely, "as an aid for treating debilitated horses when an improvement in weight, haircoat, or general physical condition is desired." Debilitation is not uncommon following disease or injury or even overwork, and anabolics will improve the general condition of these animals by improving their appetites but must be accompanied by a well-balanced diet and proper feeding.

Because anabolics are related to sex hormones, there is always some androgenic activity. There is one side effect and one disclaimer associated with them. The side effect is the reason for their abuse: overaggressiveness in some animals. If this occurs, the manufacturer states, "additional injections should not be administered."

The disclaimer reads, "In the absence of data . . . on stallions, on pregnant mares, and teratogenicity on the offspring, the drug should not be used in these animals."

⟨∞⟩

Back to Barnyard Bimbo. That fall, two years after leaving the track and receiving her last injection of the anabolic agent, she stopped fighting the teaser, preferring to just avoid him, although she was still aggressive with other mares. The following February, after a winter under lights, she responded very slightly to the teaser, and although it was still not possible to spec or palpate her, her resistance was not quite as violent.

A nearby farm had stocks they used for palpation. It's a wooden enclosure only slightly larger than a mare and there is no room to kick. Sam asked if we could use it for Bimbo, and he vanned her there, where I was able to both spec and palp her, even though she still thought little of it. Her ovaries were smallish and produced only little activity, but by May had enlarged and were producing what felt like normal follicles.

Standing for a stallion was something else, however. She kicked and reared and fought all the way, but eventually a breeding shed crew with a lot of heart got her bred. She conceived, much to my surprise. She was then ten, and Bob, trying to recoup some of his expenses of the previous three years, put her in the November sale. Both Sam and I thought he was making a mistake, especially when she brought only $16,000.

The last time I saw Bimbo it was just before the sale. She was still tough, but mellowing, and I assume she eventually became close to normal. Bob had another mare he brought to Sam's farm a few years later (her name was Shane's Pride, but the first time I heard it I wrote it down as "Schoen's Pride"), and he was there one day when I was checking her. I asked if he knew anything about Barnyard Bimbo's production record. He told us she had had three more foals by the time she was sixteen, but none thereafter.

Anabolic steroids are now restricted substances—each use must be reported—because of their abuse by human athletes and bodybuilders, but the moral is, of course, use drugs as they are intended.

I was going to end this story with praise for the languages of Polynesia—how they pronounce every letter and none are silent and none are added—even though they apparently found a special on vowels when they went to buy letters (Papeete, Kahoolawe, Kauai, Hawaii, etc.).

But then I remembered Pago Pago, which, for some reason, is pronounced "Pango Pango." Where'd they find those *n*'s? Maybe it was named by a Polish explorer.

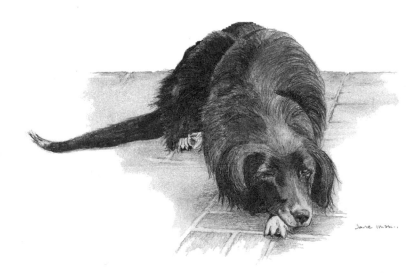

PART THREE

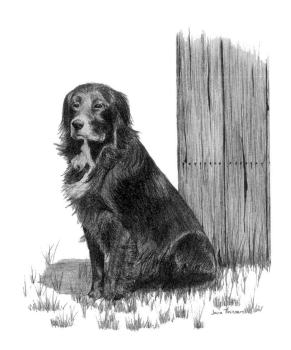

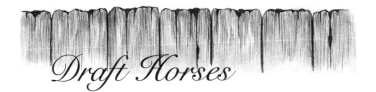

Draft Horses

I HAVE ALWAYS THOUGHT draft horses were neat, although I'm not sure why because I was in my thirties before I ever saw a real one. As a kid, I saw one in a movie and I saw pictures of them in magazines, but I never saw one in the flesh. Still, I thought they were neat.

The first real ones I saw were, believe it or not, at a large, famous theme park in Florida. The American Association of Equine Practitioners annual meeting was being held in Miami Beach, and we decided to go a few days early and take the kids to this park, then drive on down to the convention.

For transportation in the park, there were horse-drawn trolleys, and these horses were draft horses. They were beautiful and they were huge! Of the two in harness our first morning there, one must have stood 18 hands and probably weighed close to a ton. The other was maybe 17 hands and 1,600 pounds. The Thoroughbreds I work with are about 16 hands and 1,200 pounds, so these two guys dwarfed them.

And as I always believed, they were neat.

The smaller one, though, was laboring. While the trolley was stopped so passengers could get off and on, I approached the horse. He had been working, of course, pulling the trolley full of people up and down the street repeatedly, but even considering that, his respiration was very rapid and labored.

I guess I'm a vet first and a tourist second. I counted his respirations. There are breed differences and the only breed I'm fully acquainted with is the Thoroughbred, which has a resting respiratory rate of ten to twelve a minute. I imagine draft horses' resting respiratory rate is lower, maybe eight to ten, but that was secondary because this big guy sure wasn't resting. His rate was thirty-six. Thirty-six in a Thoroughbred, even after exercise, would be worrisome.

I measured his pulse. There is a place on a horse's jaw where this can be felt easily with the fingertips. The pulse in a resting Thoroughbred should be in the thirties, maybe forty. In a draft horse, I thought maybe twenties or low thirties would be normal, but, again, this big fellow was not at rest. His was nearly sixty.

And he was sweating heavily. It was a nice warm morning, but certainly not hot—maybe 70 degrees.

My wife and kids were being very patient while I did this. The trolley was ready to go again, and it took off down the street.

"Let's go, Dad," my son urged.

"Hang on, kid," I said. "I want to see something."

The other trolley, pulled by the larger horse, was coming in. Put a couple of big ears and a long nose on this guy and he could pass for an elephant. He was gigantic!

I measured his respiratory and pulse rates—twenty-four and thirty-eight. He was sweating, too, but nothing like the other one.

I realize there are differences in fitness levels. Put me in a race with Sebastian Coe and I promise you will see a vast difference in our vital signs at the finish line (assuming I get there). The big one could well have been more fit than the smaller one, or the smaller one could have been ill. In either event, the smaller one had no business working this long and this hard. It worried me.

By this time, my family's eagerness to get on with our vacation was being voiced. Both kids were begging me to get on with what we came there to do, but I told them it would be just another minute or two. My wife muttered, "It better be."

The big boy's trolley pulled out and the first one returned. I told the trolley driver of my findings and concern.

"He's okay," he said.

"But he's not," I protested. "He needs to get out of harness and be examined fully."

"He'll be through in three hours. He's okay."

Further conversation brought only further assurances that the horse was okay. Finally I asked, "Who's in charge of the animals?"

He told me where to find a fellow named Tommy and, amid loud protests from my family, I went to see him. I explained my concerns, findings, and credentials ("I'm an equine veterinarian," which impressed him as much as if I had said, "I'm a garden snail").

"He's okay," Tommy told me unemotionally. "He's only got about three hours left. I'll check him."

My family was approaching mutiny, and my wife assured me I'd done all I could do, so we went off and had fun.

It was several hours before we returned to Main Street, and there were two new horses in harness. They, too, were beautiful and both were about the size of the morning's smaller one. Against the wishes of my wife and kids, I measured the pulse and respiratory rates of these two. Both were about the same as the big horse's.

The theme park is not to be taken lightly (or quickly) when you have an eight-year-old and a six-year-old. One day is simply not enough.

On our second morning there, we went to the trolleys so I could see how the horse was doing. He wasn't there. The big one was, but the other one was one I hadn't seen the day before. And the one I was looking for wasn't there that afternoon, either.

On our third morning there (by this point we had spent at least two years of our kids' college tuition), the horse of concern was not there again. I asked the trolley driver about him.

"He's okay," he told me.

"Why hasn't he been used the last two days?" I asked.

He shrugged. "Gettin' a day or two off, I guess. I could use a day off myself."

I hope the horse was "okay." We were off to Miami Beach the next day.

It was two years later when I next came upon draft horses. Our neighbor kept two for a short time for a friend, and while he had them on his farm I was called on to vaccinate them. They were a matched pair of dappled-grey mares, each taller than 17 hands and probably weighing 1,800 pounds. They were glorious.

Then a year after that, a fellow from church called one evening. He knew who I was, but I guess I had never met him; it took five minutes of explanation before I knew who he was. I acknowledge my inability to meet people as a problem, but acknowledging it and being able to do something about it are two different things.

When it was finally cleared up as to who he was—his name was Shel—he said, "I bought a mare and foal a few weeks ago and the foal is limping."

I went there the next day. Shel owned a cattle farm, it turned out, and he had no facilities for horses, but he had the mare and foal sequestered in a tobacco barn. A *big* tobacco barn.

He met me at the barn and explained why he had bought the horses. "I think they'll look pretty in the field with the cattle." There are worse reasons for horse ownership, I guess.

To be honest, and to show what a sheltered life I lead, when a person says "mare and foal" to me, I assume what is meant is a Thoroughbred broodmare and her foal. It's kind of a tunnel vision thing associated with the Thoroughbred industry. But when he opened the door of the tobacco barn, there were definitely no Thoroughbreds in there. Standing there was a colossal bay draft mare and her equally colossal bay foal.

"Man, they're beautiful!" I exclaimed. "How old is that baby? She's enormous."

"The man I bought them from said she was about five months old and that was a few weeks ago. She started limping about three days ago and it's getting worse."

At that point, the filly, which had just been standing there, took three or four steps. She was pretty gimpy in the left foreleg. From the distance I was from her—thirty to forty feet—it looked as if it was probably in the foot.

The mare had on a halter; her foal didn't.

"Okay," I said, "put a halter on her and we'll check it out. It looks like it's her foot."

"I don't have a halter for her."

"We have to hold her so I can look at her foot."

"I was afraid of that," he said. "We can't catch her. She's never been touched."

"You have a half-grown horse there the size of a Sherman tank and she's never been touched? How in the world do you expect me to treat her?"

He looked very innocent as he replied. "Gee, you're the vet. I thought you'd know what to do."

If you've never seen a six-month-old draft horse foal, I'll describe her. Picture a 1958 Buick. Without power steering.

And if you've never seen a six-month-old draft horse foal that's never been handled, I'll describe that. Picture the '58 Buick in low gear with the emergency brake off and no driver. Except the Buick can't kick.

I wasn't sure what to do. My first inclination was to leave, but I felt an obligation to the foal. She was obviously hurting pretty badly. But I felt an obligation to my family, too; I felt obliged to stay alive so I could go on contributing to their financial needs. An unhandled foal this big could certainly affect that.

But as I said, I did feel an obligation to the foal to at least *try* to determine what was causing her lameness.

I tried to approach the filly but she was intent on maintaining at least twenty feet between us.

"I don't want to touch you, filly," I told her. "I just want to get close enough to look."

She either didn't care what I wanted to do or didn't find my voice at all reassuring—I suspect both—and she continued to hobble away.

I told Shel to help me try to get her in a corner. We got her in one, and I moved in a little closer, but she bolted and I was still unable to get a look at her foot.

"Can the mare be handled?" I asked.

"Oh, sure. She's fine."

"Okay. Get a shank and I'll try to use her as a shield. Maybe I can get closer then."

"Get a what?" he asked blankly.

Not only did he not have a shank, he didn't even know what one was, so I took the mare by the halter and tried to maneuver her sideways toward her foal. I wanted to keep her between me and her baby.

It worked. I was able to look under the mare and see the filly's foot. There was a swelling at the coronet and a little hole in it, which would soon erupt and allow the pus inside to escape. Then the foot would feel much better. This is a common condition known as gravel.

But as a precaution, she needed a tetanus vaccination. I had the owner hold the mare, and I pushed her closer to her foal. Pushing 1,800 pounds is tough; fortunately, the mare was agreeable.

With the mare pushed right against the filly, I reached around behind the mare to the foal's rump because I knew if she saw me or my hand she would run in spite of her mom's presence.

To properly administer a vaccine, you should make sure you have not placed the needle in a vein. This wasn't possible here, of course. I reached around the mare and jabbed the filly in the rump as fast as I could, injecting as I did.

The filly did two things, but she did them so fast I'm not sure which was first. She kicked—hard—and ran. The kick missed and she was gone, but vaccinated.

That's been years now and I've never been asked to go back there. When I see Shel at church, he always turns away. People are funny. His farm is on a road I travel almost daily, and I've seen the mare and her filly out in the field with the cattle hundreds of times. The filly is as big as her dam now and looks a whole lot like her. (Shel was right; they do look pretty out there among the cattle.) I can tell them apart easily; the filly still has no halter on. And every time I see them, I hope nothing ever happens to her that requires a vet's attention. She's well beyond the Buick stage now.

My last—or most recent, I should say—draft horse contact occurred in the breeding season following the above incident.

Laurie had been offered a free mare named Bet Em Big, arranged by a friend of hers who worked on another farm. Bet Em Big was twenty-one years old and hadn't had a foal since she was ten. Why they had kept her for so long I didn't understand, but maybe it was because she had produced four foals and all four had been stakes winners (one had earned nearly a half-million dollars). Patience eventually gave out, I guess, so they either had to find a home for her or put her down. Too many people send this kind of mare to a dog food company, where they can get a few cents a pound for her.

Laurie had wanted a mare for a long time. She had really wanted Princess of Kali, but I vetoed that because of my relationship with her owner. She approached me about Bet Em Big and asked if I would check her out. I told her there was little point; a mare that had been barren for eleven years was a lost cause.

"Please," she pleaded.

So I did. There was no apparent problem, but if I could get a nickel for every mare that was barren with no apparent problem, I could buy my own major-league baseball team. And stock it with free agents.

Laurie really wanted her. I reminded her that she didn't make enough money to pay a stud fee if a miracle happened and she did get in foal. I knew because I wrote her check each week.

"I have that all figured out," she smiled. "I'll give half of her to you and you can supply the stud fee!"

It was important to her, and I was confident there would be no stud fee to pay because Bet Em Big would never get in foal, so I agreed. We'd try her for one breeding season; if she didn't conceive, she had to go. Laurie agreed. All it would cost me, I was sure, was a little feed and some pasture space.

Well, Bet Em Big got in foal. This happens often enough so there always seems to be a taker for an old problem mare, but in the majority of cases the old barren mare just gets older and stays just as barren. But no one brags about those. *Everybody* hears about the successes.

Laurie was ecstatic. I was pretty pleased, too, even if I did have a $5,000 stud fee to pay. Bet Em Big had a normal but lengthy pregnancy, finally delivering a nice, big, healthy colt after 360 days of gestation.

The old girl, now twenty-two, came through the delivery in apparently fine shape. We turned them out a little on that first day, and she ran and kicked up her heels like a two-year-old. The colt was right with her.

The next morning when Laurie went to feed, Bet Em Big was trembling. She called me—I hadn't left the house yet—and I went to the barn to see what was going on.

I opened the stall door and stepped in. Bet Em Big was shaking severely. "What's wrong, old girl?" I said, and she dropped dead. Later, on the postmortem exam, we learned that she had ruptured a uterine artery and hemorrhaged, bleeding to death. This happens often enough in older mares to where it's not a big surprise.

Now we had a day-old colt and no mare. The nurse mare business here in central Kentucky is a big one. When a valuable foal is orphaned, a surrogate mother is needed, and there are farms that supply these surrogates. The nurse mare's own foal is given away or sold cheaply, and the new owner raises it on a bottle or bucket—it's a lot of work and sometimes not successful—and the nurse mare is leased to the person who needs a milk supply for his orphaned foal. Every year I have one or two clients who need one. The cost of a nurse mare lease is seven hundred to a thousand dollars, but it's money well spent.

I called the nearest nurse mare operation. All of his were gone already (it was late May and the foaling season was winding down). The next guy I called was also out of mares, but he said he'd have one in a week or so when one was due to foal. We couldn't wait that long.

I called a guy sixty miles away because he was the only other nurse mare man I knew. Yes, he had one—only one—but, "you might not like her."

"Bring her," I told him.

He arrived with the mare in mid-afternoon. He opened his trailer and led out the King Kong of nurse mares: a huge palomino draft mare!

"If you don't like her, I'll understand," he told me. "Not many people ever want one this big."

"Oh, no. She's beautiful. I love her," I replied. And besides, we had no choice. We needed a milk source and we needed it now.

The colt hadn't nursed for six to eight hours at this point, and it took very little effort to get him to nurse the big mare. And she readily accepted him. (That's not always the case. Frequently it takes hours or even days before a nurse mare accepts the strange foal, and extreme care must be taken to prevent the mare from injuring the foal.)

The nurse mare man called the mare Blondie, but she had feet the size of dinner plates, so we called her Bigfoot. I have never seen feet that big on a horse.

Bigfoot was great. She was kind and gentle and intelligent and raised her adopted son very well. When it came time to wean him, she acted just as mares act when their natural-born foals are weaned. We missed her when we returned her to her owner.

The colt grew well, and we sold him as a yearling for $27,000—not great but good enough, especially for Laurie. I took a little out of her share for sales expenses, but she ended up with more than $12,000. I didn't do as well; the stud fee, the nurse mare, the feed, and all the incidentals all worked to reduce my share to about $3,500.

The colt was named Big and Brash by his new owner, and both Bet Em Big and Bigfoot would have been proud of him if they had known about his racing career. He won a small stakes race at three and placed in a couple at four and retired at five with earnings of nearly $110,000. Bet Em Big ended up with five foals and five stakes winners. There aren't many like that.

I have not had any draft-horse patients for many years now, but I look forward to the next one. As I said, they're neat.

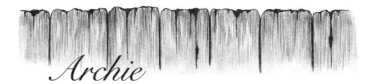

Archie

I MET TOMMY THE FIRST DAY I tried to be a veterinarian in Kentucky, and now more than twenty years later, he's still a friend and client.

I told Richard I was leaving his practice and he wished me luck. I worked on for a couple of weeks while we organized our things. All we knew was that we were headed for central Kentucky so I could work on horses.

In truth, I thought it wasn't a totally blind move, even though it turned out to be. I knew a man who lived in Versailles, a few miles west of Lexington, and he used to own a few racehorses. He was older—nearly seventy—and had been out of racing for a number of years, but he told me he had spoken with his former trainer and the trainer said he would give me a little work. I figured it was a start.

The moving van came early on a Friday morning, and it was a *slow* crew. We weren't able to get away until nearly 1 P.M. It was about five hundred miles and that would, in most cases, be a pretty easy one-day drive, but we had two kids—our son was three and our daughter five months—and two dogs and a cat, so we drove about halfway and stopped for the night. There was really no rush; no job was waiting and the moving people said our things wouldn't be there until Tuesday. They were apparently taking the scenic route.

We arrived in Lexington around noon on Saturday, checked into a motel, bought a local paper, and began looking for houses for rent. Two babies, two dogs, and a cat could coexist in a motel room for only a short period before insanity would set in, and as I would be gone most of the time, the one to go over the edge would be my wife. She insisted that we find a house ASAP.

We were lucky. There were several rentals listed, and the third one we looked at suited our needs so we took it, even though it would still be a few days before we could move in.

Sunday was spent looking around the area, and Monday I left my wife with the care of the kids and critters and went, first, to the local veterinary supplier and bought minimal supplies: a few drugs, some syringes and needles, a few implements. Then I headed out to a large Thoroughbred training center, where the man I knew had said his ex-trainer stabled his horses.

There were only two barns at the training center, but what barns they were: three hundred stalls each—ten aisles of thirty stalls—under one roof. The man I was looking for was named Nibs Beverly, but I had no idea where to find him.

I walked into one of the barns. There were horses everywhere. A young man walked by, and I asked him if he knew where I could find Nibs Beverly. He never heard of him.

I entered one of the aisles of stalls. As I stood there by the first stall, one of the biggest men I've ever seen came out of it. He wasn't that tall—maybe six-one—but he was six-one in all directions. He had to weigh at least 350 pounds. He was enormous!

"Hi," he said. "You a vet?"

"Yeah. How'd you know?"

"You look like a vet. I've never seen you around."

"I've never been around."

He introduced himself: Tommy Williams.

I told him my name and said I was looking for Nibs Beverly.

"Beverly!? What in hell you want with that no-good bum?"

I told him I'd been told that he'd give me some vet work.

Tommy laughed. "Yeah, he'll give you work." He paused and laughed again. "But he won't pay. He don't even pay his help half the time."

Rats, I thought. Now what will I do? "But my friend said . . ."

"It don't matter what your friend said. Beverly's a bum. Stay away from him."

I thanked him and turned to go.

"Wait a minute," he said. "John needs some horses wormed. You wanna do it?"

"Sure. Who's John?"

"He's the trainer I work for. John Thurlow. He'll pay. Sometimes he's slow, but he'll pay." He turned away from me and shouted, "Hey, John!"

A slender, stoop-shouldered, middle-aged man stepped out of a tack room.

Tommy called to him. "This here's Doc Kendall. I'm gonna have him worm those new horses."

"Where's Doc Marietti?" John asked.

"I ain't seen him. He's late gettin' here again and they need to be done."

So John said to go ahead. I wormed four horses that had just arrived from a farm. After we finished, Tommy said, "Before you do anything for anybody here, check with me. There's some sorry SOBs around here and you don't want nothin' to do with any of 'em. And check with us each day. John's always got somethin' to do."

I thanked him and turned to go.

"Wait a minute," he said. "Go see Charlie Tucker over in the other barn. Aisle B. Tell him I said to give you some work."

I thanked him again and went to see Charlie. He laughed and shook his head when I told him Tommy had sent me, but he had me take blood samples from two horses for Coggins tests.

When I finished, a pretty young woman came up to me. "Are you a vet? My husband told me to find one. He has a lame filly."

I asked her what her husband's name was and where I could find him, then told her I'd be right back. I ran over to find Tommy. "How's Henry Johnson?" I asked.

"Henry's okay. He ain't much of a trainer, but he's good pay. And his wife's kinda cute."

I soon found out the deadbeats and scoundrels all waited for new vets because the old ones knew them and refused to do their work, and each time someone I didn't know approached me I'd check him out with Tommy and I got burned far less often than the other new guys. And he'd refer trainers to me from time to time. In a short time, I had a busy (but not thriving) practice at the training center.

One day Tommy wasn't around when a trainer I didn't know had a horse with a pretty bad colic. The horse needed help and no other vet was available, so I treated it. Later, I told Tommy I had treated a horse for Eddie Hunter.

"You'll never see your money," he told me. "You'll end up going to the Racing Commission, but he'll lie and they won't make him pay."

It was only $45, but at that time $45 was important.

"Here's what you do," Tommy went on. "Go in his tack room and take a saddle. Let him know you got it and tell him he can have it back when he pays you."

I didn't. Then. I billed Hunter three months and never received a cent. When I went to see him about it, he was never available. Finally, I took a saddle—a real nice one; it must have been worth $350—and told him about it.

He was irate! He would have my license! I'd never work on a horse of his again! (He was right on that point.) But finally, after he finished ranting, he paid me—I insisted on cash—and I returned the saddle.

Eventually, a few of the trainers who also had farms began asking me to do their work there, too. Henry Johnson was one of the first; he had a farm with his two brothers, and they owned or boarded about twenty mares.

I would do the farms after I finished at the training center, which was usually after 11 in the morning. One day, Tommy asked, "You need help with the farm work? I'm done here by 11 or 12 every day. I can go with you and help."

I thanked him but said I couldn't possibly afford an assistant. He said he didn't want to be paid, he just thought it would be fun and it would give him something to do in the afternoons.

Riding together, I learned a lot about Tommy. I really knew nothing before.

He was a year younger than I, hadn't finished college, wasn't married and had never been, lived with his mother, and had two brothers. One brother, Robby, was some sort of sales executive and lived with his family down in Nashville or Knoxville—I've never been sure which; the other, Martin, worked in some office capacity for an oil company in Alaska.

To attempt to repay Tommy for his help, we invited him to dinner a few times. Then one day he invited us to have dinner with him and his mother. I had not met her before, but when I did, I saw there was no denying he was her child. She, too, was huge, and the two had essentially identical facial features. Later I met his two brothers. I assume there was some paternal input into the makeup of these men, but it certainly wasn't evidenced externally.

Tommy was extremely intelligent, very insightful and sensitive, and a deep thinker, but in spite of these attributes—or perhaps because of them—he was somewhat of a societal misfit. He couldn't (or wouldn't) hold a normal job, he didn't date—women just didn't like him, I came to learn (my wife, among the most tolerant of all people, said that he "scared" her)—and he even had very few male friends. He liked horses and knew about them, and that was about the extent of his interests and abilities.

Tommy's mother was on a fixed income and Tommy made next to nothing as a groom, so life was not easy for them. But Martin, the brother in Alaska, earned more money than he could spend. I understand that there are people who have that problem—professional athletes, rock stars, etc.—but it has never been one of mine.

And evidently Martin was a good son and brother. He bought a small farm for Tommy and their mom. It was only twelve acres, but it had a nice little brick house and a solid ten-stall barn, and it was fenced for horses.

Then Martin bought a broodmare for Tommy. Or I should say, gave Tommy the money to buy one for himself. She wasn't a good mare, but she was okay. Bred to the right level of stallion, she could—and did—produce foals that were profitable enough to justify the feed bills. Tommy was in the horse business.

He placed ads in the various racing industry publications and picked up a few boarders. Normally this is hard to do, but his board rates were far less than most. He wasn't getting rich, but the operation was self-supporting. He did all the work himself, so there was no payroll; and Martin had paid for the farm outright, so there was no mortgage. Feed and a modest stud fee for his mare were the only expenses.

After a couple of years, Martin came down from the frozen north for a visit. With him he had a four-month-old German Shepherd puppy. He had given the pup to his wife several weeks earlier as a third anniversary present, but he woke up one morning to find a note telling him she was gone and wouldn't be back. (She was right. He never saw her again.) He didn't think he could properly care for a puppy, so he brought him to Tommy.

The pup's name was Archduke Something von Someplace (Tommy told me, but I don't remember), but he was called simply Archie.

Tommy had never had a dog before, and he said he didn't want this one, but he fell in love with Archie in no time. They became inseparable—Tommy went nowhere without Archie. One day his mother said to me, "I believe he thinks more of that dog than he does of me." I don't know if she was right, but I would have hated to see it put to a test.

Archie grew to be a huge dog. A lot of Shepherd owners claim to have 100-pound dogs, but in truth a big Shepherd is about 80 pounds. (It's some sort of ego thing: Shepherd owners claim 100 pounds, Chihuahua owners claim 2 pounds. The Shepherd owners are closer to correct; their dogs are overestimated by 20 to 30 percent. The Chihuahua owners underestimate by 100 to 200 percent.) Archie, however, was at least 100 pounds.

And he was gentle and good-natured. He loved to play. Whenever I was there, he would bring me a stick or a ball, and as long as I would throw, he would fetch. He loved it when I brought one of the kids with me. And he was a great watchdog. I don't think he would have ever attacked or harmed anyone, but when a dog that size is barking at you, you aren't inclined to test him.

To put it rather bluntly, Tommy had no life other than the horses and Archie, and the horses couldn't sleep with him. I don't believe anyone ever loved a dog more. And I think Archie felt the same way about him. At times, it was hard for Tommy to work with the horses because Archie was always right at his side. And Tommy always carried a few dog biscuits in his pocket; he'd give two or three to Archie every time I was there.

When Archie was about five, Mrs. Williams became very ill—some sort of cancer. She didn't last long; in a matter of weeks she was gone. The bond between Tommy and Archie grew even stronger because now Archie was Tommy's *only* companion. I never saw it, but I could picture Tommy sitting around in the evenings talking to Archie.

When Archie was about eight, one day I noticed he was not walking quite right with his hind legs. I mentioned it to Tommy.

"Yeah, I know," he said. "One of the horses must've kicked him."

I knew better. Hip dysplasia is so common in German Shepherds that it's a rare dog in which it doesn't develop. In fact, at his age Archie was probably a little late in showing signs. I told Tommy of the possibility, but he said he was sure that wasn't the problem.

But it was. Hip dysplasia is progressive and Archie found it harder to get around all the time. By the time he was nine, he was almost unable to use his right hind leg and the left was weakening. A few months later he couldn't use it, either. His front legs were still fine and strong, so Tommy held his rear end up by his tail and Archie would walk alongside him using only his front legs, the useless hind legs dangling under his body.

Several times I told Tommy it wasn't fair to Archie to let him go on like that. He'd always agree with me, but then he'd change the subject.

One day when I was there to check a mare, a big hole had been dug next to the barn. Tommy, holding Archie up by his tail, was there waiting for me.

"What's with the hole?" I asked.

Tommy blinked a couple of times. I noticed his eyes were a little red. His voice cracked as he said, "Archie's ten years old today. He's the best friend I've ever had."

I knew what was coming and I wasn't sure I could do it.

"Will you please put him out of his pain?" he asked. His eyes were watering. "You're his friend. I don't want a stranger to do it."

It was for the best. I knew that, but it didn't make it any easier. The old boy had a stick in his mouth and he offered it to me, but he hadn't been able to fetch for a long time. I took it and tossed it gently back to him so he could catch it. Tommy took the stick, pulled a dog biscuit from his pocket, and gave it to Archie.

I had a hard time seeing his vein through the tears that formed in my eyes. Archie lay there patiently until I finally found it. I injected the euthanasia solution and the old dog looked up at Tommy for the short second just before he could no longer see.

Tommy sat there on the ground for a minute or so, holding his lifeless friend. I couldn't watch; I turned away and fiddled with things in the car. A veterinarian needs to be made of sterner stuff.

I helped push the dirt over the old dog. We never did check the mare that day.

That's been a few years now. Tommy still has his mare, although she's now a pensioner, and still boards a few others. He lives alone and watches a lot of TV. He has never once mentioned Archie's name (to me anyway) since that last day, but sometimes when I'm there I notice a dog biscuit or two lying where the hole had been dug.

I've asked several times if he wants another dog—I could get one for him easily—but he always says "No" and his eyes blur a little. I worry about him.

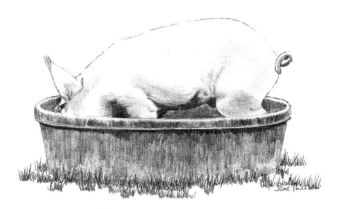

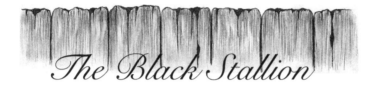

The Black Stallion

EVERYONE WHO OWNS A RACEHORSE—everyone who ever has and everyone who ever will—wants—hopes for, dreams for—a top stakes winner that goes on to be a top sire. They may not admit it, but deep down that's what they want.

Sure, some may say they just like horses, they like the sport, they just want to have a little fun—any of a number of reasons—but, in truth, everyone wants a top stakes winner that goes on to be a top sire. It's a vicarious sort of thing, I think, especially the sire part.

It's also the dream of money—big, big money. Horseracing has reached the point where a truly outstanding horse can earn eight to nine million dollars in two to three years. (Heck, not even many baseball players do that.) Dropping down from the truly outstanding to the merely really great, this kind of horse can make several hundred thousand to a few million.

And a top sire has the potential to earn additional millions in stud fees or in syndication. It's an amazing business.

This is the dream that gets people in the sport. These are the horses people read about. Generally, though, a large initial investment is required. A top racing prospect may bring a half million to more than a million dollars as a year-ling, but there is the occasional horse that sells for $5,000 or $10,000 or even $50,000—a good chunk of money to be sure, but not an unimaginable amount—that goes on to a brilliant racing career. These are the dream horses, the ones that *really* get the ink, the ones that make people want to own their own Cinderella. No matter that fewer than 2 percent ever win stakes and then only perhaps one one-hundredth of those become acclaimed as "great." Hope springs eternal.

Of course, very little is ever written about the million-dollar yearling that never wins a race or the $400,000 one that gets hurt and never even *runs* a race.

Newcomers interested in owning a racehorse and who aren't familiar with the ins and outs of horses and the horse business should seek advice from someone who is (see the chapter "Buyer Beware"), but frequently they don't and the result is often disaster. And other times—or at least *one* other time—the neo-phyte horseman's requirements for a potential racehorse preclude professional advice.

There are more bad horses than good ones. I guess there are more bad any-things than good ones—people, dogs, kangaroos, petunias, you name it. By "bad," I don't mean evil. I mean discredits to their species as performers.

People have asked me from time to time if I ever work on any "good" horses and, of course, they mean top performers.

Well, yes, I do, but their stories are generally not as interesting, and any-how, if they're *really* good, they've already received plenty of ink. And too, as I said, there are a whole lot more bad (or at least, not good) horses out there.

But over the years there have been good horses under my care. As I no longer do track work, there are no current stakes performers I work on, but years ago I was the vet for a Kentucky Derby runner-up. Fortunately for his owner and trainer, he was sound and all I had to do was worm and vaccinate him. And there were several other good stakes horses at one time or another.

Also, I have given early care to a number of foals that went on to glory on the track and to their dams on the farm, but few of their stories are worth the effort to put on paper.

One good horse, though, is worthy of mention.

A client—a woman named Charlene—had a farm on which she boarded several mares. Her brother, Charlie, a businessman who knew nothing about horses but enjoyed going to the races, was a frequent visitor to the farm. Eventually, he decided he wanted to own a racehorse of his own.

He talked to Charlene about it. She suggested to him that he attend the yearling sales and buy one there; she also said that he should have me help him.

One day at the farm he approached me about it. Sure, I said, I'd be glad to examine any yearling in which he had an interest. "How much do you want to spend?" I asked.

"Seventy-five hundred max," he answered. "I should be able to get a stakes winner for that."

Uh-oh, I thought, we're in trouble. I tried to tell him that just because he *wanted* a stakes winner, the chances were pretty good—*very* good—that he would not get one.

"He'll need to be. I want to stand him at stud," he explained, matter-of-factly.

Oh, boy. "So you're going to buy a colt?"

"A stallion. I want a black stallion."

As the conversation progressed, if that's what you call the direction in which it was going, it was determined that his criteria were only color, sex, and price: a black colt ("stallion") for no more than $7,500. Pedigree and conformation were secondary. I told him that he didn't need me; his sister could find one for him and he wouldn't have to pay her as he would me.

Sure enough, at the September yearling sales in Lexington she bought him a "black stallion" for $5,500. I first saw the colt a few days later at the farm. He was officially "dark bay or brown" (a Thoroughbred registered as "black" is very rare), but he didn't miss black by much, and he wasn't a bad-looking individual at all. The pedigree was borderline, at best—the nearest black type was in the second dam—but his dam had produced a couple of winners. (In a pedigree on a catalog page, stakes winners' names are printed in boldfaced type; hence, the term *black type*. "Second dam" means the granddam on the dam's side.) Charlie *loved* him. He immediately named him Dandy Decision.

His sister was not too happy with the colt, however. "He's nasty," she said. "He bites and strikes and won't get caught. I'll be glad when he leaves to be broken."

He did, in early October. She related his progress to me periodically—he was still mean as a snake and getting increasingly more dangerous to work around. One day when her brother was at the farm, she told me of a particularly nasty incident: Dandy Decision, now two, had seriously bitten his hot walker.

"Sounds like he needs to be cut," I said.

"Cut?" said Charlie. "What's that?"

"Gelded," I explained. "It'll improve his disposition."

The guy visibly blanched. "Gelded?" he gulped. "You mean . . ." He appeared to be searching for the words. "You mean . . . his . . . his . . . *balls?*" He blushed.

"Yes!" snapped Charlene. "He's dangerous!"

"But . . . but . . . ," stammered Charlie.

"It's okay, Charlie," his sister said. "We're talking about *his* balls, not yours."

He blushed again. "But he can't stand at stud then."

"Look, Charlie, the odds are so much against your horse being successful enough to stand at stud as to be almost unimaginable," Charlene told him.

"He's gonna be a stakes winner!" Charlie insisted. "He'll be a stud!"

Charlene and I looked at each other. She shrugged.

Dandy Decision continued to be a problem. Two of the trainer's employees quit because of him.

Many weeks later, Charlie approached me at the farm. "What's a riggling?" he asked.

"A riggling? You mean 'ridgling.' It's a cryptorchid."

"A what?"

"One testicle is undescended. Because of the heat in the abdominal cavity, the retained testicle produces a higher level of hormones and makes a ridgling even more studdish than a horse with both testes descended. A ridgling is usually very mean. Is that Dandy's problem?"

"That's what the trainer says."

"Then he *has* to be cut."

Charlie had heard this so often that he no longer recoiled from it, he just got very defensive. *"He's going to be a stakes winner and stand at stud!"* he insisted for the umpteenth time.

I explained the Jockey Club rule about standing ridglings at stud and that the condition was pretty highly inherited. Since then, I think the rule has been changed, but it still makes good sense to geld them because of the dangers involved in handling them.

"How will they know if I don't tell them?" he reasoned.

Dandy's training continued and from the reports I heard he was getting ranker by the day. He couldn't work successfully with other horses because he preferred to savage them rather than run. (*Savage* is a racetrack term for biting another horse.) Another employee quit. He slapped a groom in the face with a front foot and broke his nose.

Finally, though—somehow—he got to the races in June. He was a crazy horse and so intent on eating the horse and jockey next to him that he finished dead last. Three weeks later he ran again and beat one horse, but acted so badly in the starting gate that the trainer was told not to enter him again until he had been okayed again. The trainer shipped him directly to the farm and told Charlie that that was the last straw. He wouldn't train him anymore.

Charlie was morose. Charlene and I explained again the losing battle he was fighting. But "black stallion at stud" was all we heard.

Charlie sent him to another trainer, who returned him in less than a month. "I don't need horses that much," the trainer told him.

Finally, Charlene's employees refused to work with Dandy, just after I refused one day to worm him. "Life's too short as it is," I told her.

Charlene told Charlie the horse had to go, so at last, Charlie consented to have him gelded. He came to realize that Dandy would never win a race if he couldn't be trained. We sent him to a local clinic where the surgery was performed. Ninety days later he was a different horse and went back into training with his original trainer.

Dandy Decision raced until he was seven or eight and won seven stakes and nearly $400,000 along the way. At the end, he was still running in allowance races. He wasn't a great horse, but he sure was a good one.

Charlie talked forever about what a great stud his "black stallion" would have been. He never forgave Charlene or me for "ruining" him. "I never should have listened to you," he told us every time Dandy ran and for years after his retirement.

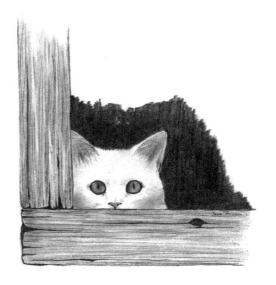

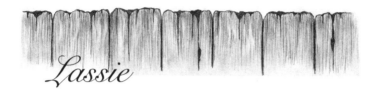

Lassie

THIS STORY IS PRETTY HOKEY-SOUNDING. I won't try to explain it or interpret it; I'll just relate the facts as I saw and heard them.

Sharon Maysfield today is a veterinarian in Pennsylvania, or was the last time I heard, but she grew up around here. She was an only child and a late arrival at that. Her mother told me once that she and Sharon's father were in their early forties and had been married nearly twenty years when Sharon was born and they had long since stopped hoping for a child. None of this has anything to do with the story, but I include it because there's probably a useful moral here: Never give up.

I first met Sharon when she was fifteen. Her horse—the family's only horse—was colicking and she couldn't reach her regular vet. It was Labor Day, I think, but it was so long ago that I won't swear to it now. I do recall it *was* a cookout type of holiday, so I guess it could have been Memorial Day or the Fourth of July.

Her horse was a Thoroughbred gelding that had failed as a racehorse. In four years of attempting to race, he had been in thirty-some races and had only one second to show for his efforts. The parent Maysfields had bought him for Sharon as a birthday present when he was five years old and she was twelve.

The owner was a man with whom Mr. Maysfield had some minor business dealings. His name was MacKenzie, but people called him "Mac." The horse, whose registered name I don't recall being told, was huge and this may have been part of the reason for his inability to run satisfactorily. It wasn't that he was particularly tall; he was about 16 hands and a couple of inches, and a lot of Thoroughbreds are that tall, but he had a massive body and gigantic, coarse bones. I would estimate his weight at 1,600 pounds. Because of his size and because of whom he was acquired from, Sharon named him Big Mac. It was an uncommonly fitting name.

But I knew none of this history that first time I went to the Maysfield's seven- or eight-acre "farm." And Big Mac really doesn't play much of a role in this story other than as the vehicle that brought me into repeated contact with the Maysfield family.

On that first trip to the farm, Big Mac had a very mild bellyache and responded readily to treatment. Sharon told me that sometimes her regular vet was hard to get in touch with and asked if I had time to tend to Big Mac on a regular basis. I told her I did and the "regular" basis turned out to be maybe six times a year until she graduated vet school some twelve years later.

When I arrived that day, I was greeted at the barn by Sharon, who was tiny (I thought she was maybe ten rather than fifteen), and a largish, long-haired dog that seemed delighted to see me. (I later learned she was delighted to see everyone.) There was also a cat—solid black with a small white spot on his forehead; I've never seen another marked like that.

The dog, named Lassie (it was pretty obvious that a Collie had entered into her gene pool at some point), and the cat, Foster, had also been birthday gifts for Sharon, Foster when she was eight and Lassie at nine. These facts, too, I learned over time.

I learned, also, that the worlds of Lassie and Foster centered on Sharon. They knew when the school bus brought her home, and they were there to greet her. They slept with her. When she began dating, they would sit by the front door awaiting her return. I saw none of this, of course; it was told to me in bits and pieces by her mother and father over the years.

When she was eighteen, Sharon went away to college, choosing, for a reason I never knew, Western Kentucky University, way out in, where else?, western Kentucky (Bowling Green, to be exact). It was so far away that it was in a different time zone (central; we're eastern here).

By now, those of you who are still reading this are probably thinking, "Is there a point to all this?" (The rest of you have undoubtedly skipped to the next chapter.) Well, we're getting there. Never give up. (See the first page of this chapter.) We're getting to the hokey part.

Sharon came home from college on the average of once a month, but the weekends varied. It may have been the second weekend one month, the third another, etc. Sometimes she would call first; more often than not, she would just show up late on a Friday evening, but her parents always knew when she was coming because of Lassie and Foster. Approximately an hour before Sharon would arrive, Lassie would sit by the front door and begin whimpering and Foster would pace back and forth by her. At first, of course, the elder Maysfields thought it was coincidence, but by the end of Sharon's freshman year they realized it was more than that.

I heard these tales usually from Mr. Maysfield, who at this point was in his early sixties and retired, on those occasions when I was there to worm or vaccinate Big Mac. I thought the stories were cute, but I suspected the Maysfields were either getting dotty or perhaps using too much cooking sherry on Friday evenings. Mr. Maysfield sometimes asked my opinion of the stories, and all I would say was, "Gosh, Mr. Maysfield, there's more to dogs and cats than we know."

This continued through Sharon's sophomore year. In fact, Sharon stopped calling altogether when she was coming home. The old dog and cat would let her parents know at least an hour before she drove in.

In her junior year, when she was twenty and Lassie eleven, I was at the Maysfield farm around 10 one morning to remove sutures from Big Mac's left hip. He had somehow acquired a long but shallow cut the week before; it wasn't even all the way through the skin but because of its length, I decided to suture it, although it may well have healed just fine without it.

As I was snipping the suture material, Mr. Maysfield asked, "Will you come up to the house and take a look at Lassie when you've finished here?"

"What's wrong with the old gal?" I asked.

"I don't know. She just lays there like maybe she's unconscious," he replied.

When I got to the house, Lassie was lying on the living room floor with her eyes closed. Curled up by her belly was Foster. I tried to rouse the old dog. I picked up her head and it dropped back to the floor. I pinched her toes to see if there was any response. There was, but it was minimal.

"What happened?" I asked. "Did you find her like this when you got up this morning?"

She had been normal earlier that day. She and Foster had gone out and made their rounds and returned to the house and wanted back in about eight o'clock.

Mrs. Maysfield told me what happened next. "About 8:30, she barked frantically four or five times—almost like she was scared—and then fell down. This is the way she's been since."

There are conditions—diseases, injuries—that can sort of do this to a dog, but none of them seemed to fit. I had no idea what was wrong with her.

"Maybe it's just the old girl's time," I suggested, but added that perhaps they should take her to someone who did a little more small-animal work than I did. They said they would. I left then; it was right at 11 o'clock.

The rest of this story is strictly hearsay, related to me a few weeks later by Mr. Maysfield.

I had been gone about five minutes when the Maysfields received a phone call. Sharon had been in an automobile accident and was in the hospital, unconscious. The accident had occurred at approximately 7:30 that morning,

Bowling Green time, but no one had called earlier because Sharon had no identification on her and the girl who had been driving couldn't tell them who Sharon was because she was also unconscious. Finally, the driver had awakened and told them Sharon's name.

The Maysfields began the long drive across the state, but first called their neighbors and friends, the Watermans, and asked that they look after the Maysfield house and animals for however long they were away.

The Watermans were also retired and Mr. Waterman came right over. He said he'd stay there until the Maysfields returned. He also said he'd take Lassie to the small-animal vet as soon as his wife, who had gone shopping, returned with the car.

Somewhere between 1:30 and 2:00, Mrs. Waterman had still not returned, but according to Mr. Waterman, Lassie rolled up on her chest, shook her head a few times, whimpered, and stood up. She had been down and out for about five hours.

The Maysfields were in transit at that point. When they finally arrived at the far-away hospital, they found Sharon awake and alert, bruised and sore and with a fractured thumb and a *big* headache but otherwise okay. She had come to at about 12:40 and had been unconscious for about five hours. She and her roommate both had suffered mild concussions.

This is what happened that morning in Bowling Green: Sharon and her roommate left their apartment a few minutes before 7:30, the roommate driving. Another car ran a stoplight from the right—Sharon's side. Sharon saw it coming and screamed, then the other car hit them. Both girls were knocked unconscious, but neither was hurt badly and the driver of the other car was uninjured. Both cars were totaled.

Every time the story was told, the Maysfields were careful to point out that 8:30 A.M. Paris time is 7:30 A.M. Bowling Green time, and 12:40 P.M. Bowling Green time is between 1:30 and 2:00 P.M. Paris time. They made sure the listener knew that. They insisted Lassie *knew,* that she *felt* what was happening to Sharon.

I can't comment because I don't know. This is the story as I saw and heard it.

Epilogue: Lassie lived to the age of fifteen and never had another "unconscious" episode. She had been doing poorly for quite a while toward the end. Sharon was in vet school in Alabama and couldn't come home very often, but she called twice a week and Mr. Maysfield told me the first thing she'd always do was ask about Lassie. The dog got to where all she'd do was go outside and eliminate and come right back in and sleep.

When Sharon came home for Christmas break in her junior year in vet school, Lassie apparently knew she was coming. She sat by the front door staring at it and wagging her tail for more than an hour before Sharon got there. She greeted the girl as she had done since she was a puppy—jumping on her, whimpering, licking her face—and that night slept with her, as always. She never woke up.

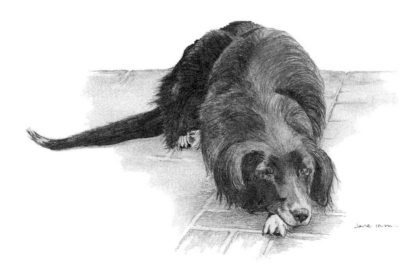

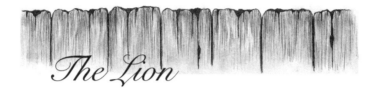

The Lion

MAYBE I SHOULD HAVE BEEN a zoo veterinarian. It never occurred to me earlier, but it may well be what I should have pursued. You see, I have vastly better animal skills than I have people skills. Perhaps in a small-animal practice that isn't as important as it is in equine practice, but it is overwhelmingly important with horse people.

The reader will recall (unless, of course, the reader hasn't read *The Animals in My Life*) that my association with Robin, Calico, and Chick was probably the point in my life when I decided I wanted to be a veterinarian. I was a very little boy then and I loved these three, although I must admit that most of my relationships with chickens from that point until today have involved the cooperation of Colonel Sanders and his ilk.

Before that, though, and indeed, as long as I can remember, I liked animals. They fascinated me. I remember my earliest books: picture books of animals. Later I had a series of small (in dimension) books—I wish I remembered what they were called—each of which was devoted to a type of animal: birds, fish, mammals of North America, insects, etc. There were pictures of each, a small amount of text describing them, and a map showing the creature's natural range.

Then there were books of dog breeds and books of horse breeds. (There may have been books of cattle breeds, but if there were I never saw them; perhaps there's a lesson there.) I read them all.

And I read *My Friend Flicka* and *The Black Stallion* and all the great horse stories. And dog stories. Anyone who can read Terhune's *Lad, A Dog* and not immediately want a Collie is an alien.

My favorite toys were a set of animals I should never have been allowed to play with. I have no idea what they cost, but if they were made today very few people could afford them. They were African mammals, all in scale to each other. The male lion, for instance, was about four or five inches long and maybe two inches tall. The gorilla was probably five inches tall.

They were made of plaster over a wire frame. I know because the plaster broke from their legs easily—too easily in the hands of a small boy—and their wire skeletons became visible.

They were beautifully painted and detailed. When friends came over, I always wanted to play "Africa," but they wanted to play with toy cars or guns or cowboys or other things that were okay but certainly weren't as much fun as playing with animals.

I destroyed that marvelous set of animals. They just could not withstand the love I bestowed on them. I must have had forty or fifty, and one by one they dropped by the wayside. I mourned them all. The giraffe was the first to go—four skinny legs and a skinny neck—and the gorilla and a lion cub lasted the longest.

Back to the importance of people skills in equine practice. I'm not a party-goer or a drinking buddy or a social climber. I don't even play golf. These are important attributes in the horse business, essentially a very small segment of society. I'd rather be home with my family when I'm not working; I'd rather play baseball with my son, take my daughter to music (herein used in its loosest sense) concerts, and go with my wife to a movie or dinner.

I was slow to realize this as a problem. I believed that competency and good service—being there when promised or needed—would suffice, but I learned in time that many horsemen, be they farm owners or managers, prefer a vet who "plays the game," even though a little may be lost in service and competency. I'm not saying an incompetent good ol' boy can make it as an equine vet—he can't; the difference may be a 3 to 5 percent smaller foal crop or one horse every five years that has to go to surgery because the vet was slow in getting to what began as a mild colic. And then, of course, there are the worst kind of vets: those who are both competent and conscientious *and* game-players.

Don't think I'm complaining, even though I may be, because I have good clients. There are horse people who are just like me—dull and mundane—and some of them own or manage a whole lot of horses and they need a vet, too.

But I really do prefer the animals to the people, and I get along with them much better, and that is why I think maybe I should have been a zoo vet. As I said, it never occurred to me. The reason I think about it now is because of an incident in a small town about twenty miles from here. The story was told to me by a friend who is a reporter for that small town's three-times-a-week newspaper. She covered the story.

It seems a couple in the county owned a lion, a full-grown male African lion. Rumor (unsubstantiated and therefore not reported) has it that this couple grew marijuana and the lion was their security system.

The lion, of course, should never have been in rural Kentucky in the first place, but he was and he got loose. A furor went up in the area, even though I'm sure the lion wanted as little to do with the local residents as he could manage, and the result, unfortunately, was a dead lion. Someone shot him. The poor lion was there not by his wishes or by his doing, but it didn't matter.

It's a sad tale, but it brought back memories of another lion, the only one I've ever been close enough to to touch. This is a happier story.

In my senior year in vet school, the nearest zoo—some eighty or so miles away—sent the school a lion that needed surgery. He had an abscessed tooth and it had to be removed.

The lion was brought over in a shipping crate just barely big enough for him to fit into. The sides, top, and bottom were solid, but each end had bars. He couldn't turn and could just barely stand.

I was on small-animal clinic duty at this time, and even though he wasn't exactly a "small" animal, he was a cat, so we were notified of his imminent arrival. When he got there, we all eagerly trotted down to the large animal receiving area, where the shipping crate was removed from the truck that had brought it.

The big boy was ticked off and I don't blame him. It was bad enough that he had an exceedingly painful tooth (he hadn't been able to eat for two days) and must have felt miserable, and he was stuck in a box unable to move, but now a couple dozen gawking idiots had surrounded him and were pointing and saying inane things. He growled a lot, made a half-hearted roar, and slapped the bars with his front feet, claws extended.

He was huge and he was beautiful. I've seen photos and movies of lions in the wild and never fully appreciated their size, and the males in the wild have small manes due, I guess, to losing hair in the tall grass and underbrush. This guy's mane was full and luxuriant. I knew people hunted them, but I remember thinking, "How could anyone kill something so magnificent?"

As I said, he was ticked off, and he became even more so—for a moment. Dr. Paulter, who was to do the surgery to remove the tooth, had approached him from the rear with what appeared to be a lethal dose of injectable anesthetic in a syringe. The syringe was attached to a long device that enabled the injection to be given while the injector himself maintained a discreet distance.

Dr. Paulter popped the lion in the back of a hind leg, evoking a roar of disapproval that would have driven the monkeys, if there had been any in the vicinity, to the highest reaches of the jungle canopy and the zebras, again assuming there had been a wild herd somewhere nearby, into a frenzied stampede across the plain. The lion jumped so hard that the cage lifted off the ground.

But then he was asleep. He was removed from the cage, his feet were bound, and an oral speculum was placed in his mouth, for two reasons: (1) it held the mouth open so Dr. Paulter could remove the tooth; and (2) it held the mouth open so the lion couldn't close it on any portion of Dr. Paulter should he awaken early.

The tooth removal itself went quickly, but infection had to be controlled, so he had to be placed on antibiotics.

If you have never done it, remember this: There is no easy way to give a cat medication. Even a soft, cuddly, adorably sweet little kitten, when you open its mouth to attempt to give it a pill, will shred you or puncture you or, most likely, both. Both claws and teeth will wreak havoc on you. The same goes if an injection is attempted.

There are, however, ways a little kitty can be overcome. There are "cat bags" into which the animal may be placed, exposing only the area needed—the head, a leg, etc. And there are little nylon gizmos with which pills may be given so you don't have to stick your finger in kitty's mouth. Fingers are hard to replace.

These were not exactly applicable to this patient, though. Even if you had a bag big enough and strong enough, getting a lion into it would be an insurmountable challenge, and I don't believe they make nylon pill deliverers in lion sizes.

Our lion was unbound and reloaded into his cage and Dr. Paulter gave him an initial dose of antibiotic via injection while he was still asleep (but rousing). The crate was put back on the truck that brought it, and the big cat was returned to his zoo home, with instructions to place his medication in his feed twice a day. It must have worked because several months later I went to the zoo and there he was, healthy and as happy as a lion can be, I guess, when he is in captivity.

He didn't remember me, of course. I was just one of the idiots who had gawked at him, but I was also the one who, while he was under anesthesia, rubbed his body and ran my hands through his mane and across his beautiful face. What a wonderful experience.

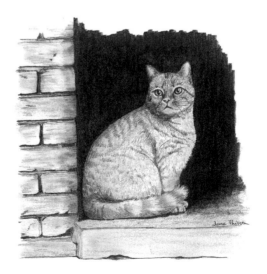

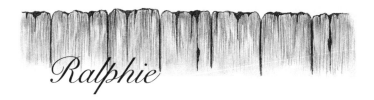

Ralphie

KIDS AND DOGS HAVE A LOT IN COMMON:

1. They both need to be housebroken.
2. They both need to be taught to stay out of the street and not to take treats from strangers.
3. They both are expensive over the years.
4. At certain times in their lives, neither can be fully trusted with members of the opposite sex.
5. They're both with us for too short a time. Dogs live way too short, kids grow up way too fast.

Of course, they have their differences, too.

1. It's cheaper, easier, and quicker to get a dog.
2. Dogs don't talk back.
3. Dogs treat you better.
4. Dogs come when they're called and do what they're told.
5. Dogs don't get embarrassed by your mere presence.

6. Left alone in the house, dogs will protect it. Left alone in the house, kids will invite friends over.

7. Dogs don't drive.

Even though the balance seems to favor dogs, most of us still have kids. Perhaps some future, enlightened society will come to realize the error in this. Of course, for the future of that society, replacement members will be needed, but being an advanced society, these replacements will be kept in storage until they are needed to enter the society in a productive manner, say, at the age of twenty-five. Life will be so much easier.

But until that day, we will continue to reproduce as we have always done, and the fruits of that reproductive process will enter our households as helpless little things who have no idea what we are saying to them, grow into helpless larger things (helpless in that they aren't capable of putting their clothes or toys away, cleaning their rooms, and things like that), who know perfectly well what we are saying to them but choose to ignore it, and finally grow into functional units who *can* put clothes away and maintain clean rooms and even understand and heed our words but immediately move out so they can go through the same process that we have been forced to endure for the past twenty-odd years.

But in spite of that, we love them, and the time they are with us is too short.

Our son finished college a short while ago. I'm not sure how. It seems as if just last week I was teaching him how to ride his Big Wheel, but somehow in that short time he grew up.

And shortly after graduation, our little boy married a woman—a full-grown adult woman who he met at college. Sure, they're the same age, but she was an *adult*—how do we know that she was ever anything but an adult?—and she just *stole* our little boy.

These two set forth in the world to earn a living. He did not become a veterinarian; he has little scientific aptitude and even less agricultural aptitude. He likes horses but could live without them. (He doesn't know if he likes cows, having never been exposed to them. I protect my kids.) He loves dogs and really, really likes cats, though.

(With the beginning of this story, I bet you think it's about a dog. It's not. Sorry.)

The young couple weren't in a position to have a dog—too much time away from home at work, small apartment, etc.—so pet ownership was put on hold. (If he needed a pet fix, he could always come home for a visit, where Bastille, our old Lab, is always delighted to see him.)

One morning, shortly after they moved into their place, a small, rough-looking orange cat was frantically scratching and meowing at their door. When the door was opened, he came in, went to a chair, curled up, and went to sleep.

After a short nap, he got up, stretched, went to the door, and scratched and meowed until he was let back out.

Scott and Susie left for work then and thought no more of the cat . . . until Susie came back home at 4:00. There he was—frantically scratching and meowing at the door. Once in, he wandered around the apartment for a few minutes and then returned to the door, scratching and meowing until she let him out again. By the time Scott got home at 5:30, this had happened three times.

They figured that the people who lived in the apartment before them must have left him when they moved or took him but he came back on his own to familiar surroundings, so they called their landlady and told her they had the previous residents' cat.

"They didn't have a cat," the landlady said.

Okay, then maybe he was a neighbor's cat. They asked the people in the apartment next door. No, they didn't own a cat. Upstairs—same. No cat.

There were seven apartments in the building and three buildings. They checked them all. Either no one owned a cat or, if they did, this one wasn't theirs.

That evening the cat came and went a half-dozen times, each time scratching and meowing at the door until it was opened for him. His last departure was after 10 and then Scott and Susie went to bed. They didn't really expect to see him again.

But when Scott got up the next morning at 5:30 the cat was there, scratching and meowing frantically to get in. He came in and took a nap and twenty minutes later he wanted back out.

And again that afternoon he was waiting when they came home. They watched him when they put him out one of the times that evening (about fifteen minutes after they had let him in), to try to see where he went. Maybe that would give a clue as to who owned him, but all he did was run across the busy street in front of the apartment buildings and disappear in the overgrown weeds in the vacant field over there.

And a short time later, he returned. This time they were having dinner—fish sticks—and the cat let them know that he wanted some, too. They gave him a few bites.

After two or three more days of this—repeated visits by the cat during which times he wanted in or out two or three times an hour—they came to the conclusion that they owned a cat. They went out and bought a cat box, cat sand, and cat food.

They needed to name him if he was going to be a permanent member of their household. Scott, for reasons even he didn't know, said he wanted to call him "Ralph." Susie didn't like that and showed a little more imagination.

"He's orange and he's rough-looking," she said, "and he likes fish. Let's call him 'Orange Roughy.'"

"What kind of name is that?" Scott wanted to know.

"It's a kind of fish. It fits him perfectly."

"I like 'Ralph,'" my less-imaginative son said.

Well, they compromised. He became "Orange Ralphie."

Ralphie settled in well, but in a few days he began scratching and meowing at inside doors, too—closet doors, room doors, pantry doors. He never met a door he didn't want to pass through. It was an easily solved problem, however; all the doors in their apartment now remain slightly ajar. The only door that needs attending is the one to the outside world.

Ralphie is a good cat. They've never found where he came from, but it doesn't matter. They're happy with him and he seems to be happy with them. It is slightly annoying, though, to know that any minute he will want to be on the other side of the door, whichever side he's on.

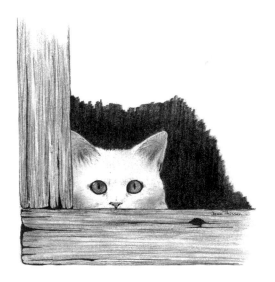

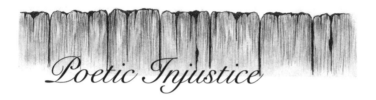

Poetic Injustice

PARTICIPATION IN HORSERACING in this country by African Americans is not great. I don't know why; I guess it goes back to economic opportunity. Fortunately, that's changing as our country gets its collective head on straight and racial equality, though not yet attained, is in sight on the distant horizon.

The limited number of blacks who participate (if that's the word) in racing is distributed much as the whites, however: Most are employed at the groom/hot-walker level, the next most as exercise riders, then jockeys, then trainers, and then a very few owners. (But no vets that I know of.) And there are a few (of all colors) who perform *all* the tasks for their one- or two-horse stables.

I don't think competence has racial limits; in fact, someone in a minority may actually strive a little harder trying to show he can hold his own. Of the few black trainers I've known, there have been a higher percentage who were as "good" (a nebulous concept) as their Caucasian peers.

(The situation is just the opposite in Jamaica, the only other country in which I'm well acquainted with the racing industry. In a nation in which 98 percent of the population is of African descent, opportunities are quite different.)

Through the years I have had a few black clients—a few trainers and a few owners. Very few. Because they are so few, they're easy to remember.

One owner was a huge, muscular man from Philadelphia named Ron, who kept his horses in Kentucky. He always dressed in exquisitely tailored, high-quality suits, and he was always accompanied by two companions: his strikingly beautiful girlfriend and his bodyguard, both of whom dressed as well as he did.

When they attended the yearling sales, his girlfriend carried a briefcase filled with cash, which he used to pay for any purchases he would make. I don't know how much money was in the briefcase, but he once bought a yearling for $88,000 and paid for it on the spot.

Unfortunately, Ron's source of income was frowned upon by some. He was in the numbers racket. (At that time it was illegal, but today most states are in the same racket; they call it the "lottery.") One afternoon I received a visit from an Internal Revenue Service agent. He asked if I knew Ron, had I done veterinary work for him, had he paid me (he sure had—by return mail, regardless of how large the bill was), did I have records, etc.

The answers to all of the agent's questions were yes, so he asked for all my records pertaining to Ron. I told him I'd been doing work for him for several years and it would be a real pain to get everything together. Being an understanding, good-humored sort, he told me if I refused to cooperate (which I hadn't), he would subpoena them.

I firmly believe that there are several creatures in this world we don't want to alienate. Grizzly bears, for instance. Cows. Disgruntled postal workers. IRS agents. So I gathered everything I had on Ron—it took a couple of days to find it all—and made copies for this guy. It was pretty straightforward stuff—bills for worming, vaccinating, medicating, etc.—and probably came to $10,000 or so over the years, not a large amount at all for a racehorse owner. Certainly none of it was incriminating, but they must have found something from some source because Ron was convicted of something and imprisoned. I think he must be out by now but I have heard nothing about him nor have I seen him at the sales.

ᑲᕼᕽ

The only other African American owners I've had for clients were both named Jim, and they were both clients at the same time. Jim-1 was apparently fairly well-off; he owned three mares and raced their offspring. He boarded them at a farm where I was the vet.

Jim-2 was a hard-working blue-collar guy who owned one mare, which he kept on a small parcel of land that he leased. He, too, raced the offspring and he did everything himself—except ride them in races. He was the stall mucker/groom/hot walker/exercise boy/trainer/owner. His wife and son were his only help, such as it was.

Jim-1 and Jim-2 knew each other, but I didn't know that for several years.

Jim-1's mares came under my care when he moved them to a client's boarding farm many years ago, and Jim-2's mare became my patient, coincidentally, the same year. Jim-1's mares had all had foals before; Jim-2's was just off the track.

Jim-1's mares were named Flo, Buttered Toast, and Peon's Poem, a very large, very coarse plain bay. The first year I worked on them, Flo and Buttered Toast were in foal, but Peon's Poem was not, although she had had a foal—her first—the previous year. Flo and Buttered Toast did everything right—foaled easily, bred easily, never got sick, raised healthy foals, etc.—so their stories are of little interest. (No one ever writes about the teenagers who *don't* get in trouble, either.)

Jim-2's mare, Carolina Ruby, was the same. She didn't get in foal that first year, but conceived the next year and then had six straight foals before she missed again. No story here, either.

But Peon's Poem was a problem mare. Problem mares are very profitable for a vet but a serious expense for their owners. And usually, if the problem remains, the mare is disposed of—sold or given away or put down. Occasionally, it's the vet who goes, in pursuance with the Broodmare Owner's Creed.

That goes something like this: If a man owns ten mares and all ten get in foal, he tells the world, "*I* got all my mares in foal!" However, if only five of the ten conceive, the word that is spread is, "That darn *vet* only got half my mares in foal!" We learn to live with it.

As I said, Peon's Poem was not in foal that first year I worked on her, and with good reason: She was dirty (a euphemism for a uterine infection). A culture showed us the causative organism and the drugs we could use to combat it, so treatment was instituted. Usually, one course of therapy will solve the problem, a follow-up culture will show no further infection, and the mare can be bred. And usually she conceives.

Peon's Poem's infection, however, was a stubborn one. That first year she was cultured and treated three times at a cost to Jim-1 of several hundred dollars. Finally, after the third treatment, we got a clean culture and she was bred.

But she didn't conceive, so we cultured her again on her next heat period. She was dirty again and again the infection was a stubborn one. She ended up barren for a second year, I ended up with a considerable amount of income from her, and Jim-1 ended up disappointed, but her first (and only, so far) foal, a yearling at this point, was a knockout, so he wasn't going to give up on her.

We continued to work on Peon's Poem through the summer and into the fall. She finally cultured clean in September and another culture in early October was also clean, so we were ready for the next breeding season.

A culture in late February was clean, too, so we bred her. Well, you know what happened: She didn't conceive and came up dirty again. (This isn't unusual in chronically infected mares. The uterine wall becomes compromised and can't withstand the normal bacterial contamination resulting from the act of mating.)

In addition to further treatment, we biopsied her uterus. There was damage which had resulted from a combination of the infections and the treatments. To shorten the narrative a little, she was barren again—for the third straight year.

In the meantime, her foal, now two, won his first two starts and then ran second in a stakes race. He looked as if he would be pretty good, so Jim-1 wanted another foal from Peon's Poem more than ever.

Well, Peon's Poem did it again the next year: dirty and barren. Four years in a row. Cultures, treatments, and the attempts to correct the damage to the uterine wall had now cost Jim-1 several thousand dollars, and that didn't include his board bills, farrier bills, and routine vet bills (vaccinations, wormings, etc.).

Her now three-year-old won a stakes race and was nominated to the Kentucky Derby (but didn't run in it; he was nowhere near that quality). His earnings were approaching $80,000 and so Jim-1 wanted to try again with Peon's Poem. I guess, as I look at this in retrospect, her foal was supporting her.

But it was the same story the next year. We'd treat her a couple times, she'd culture clean, then we'd breed her and she'd come up dirty again. In late May, her foal, now four, was injured badly and had to be retired (he had earned almost $120,000). In June, Jim-1 called me. "I've had it," he said, "I'm getting rid of Peon's Poem."

I certainly didn't blame him. She had been profitable for me over the years, but a real frustration. I have never liked it when a mare under my care comes up barren, and I like it even less when I can't correct the problem. I know it's not intentional, but even so, I take it personally.

Jim-1 acted quickly. Within three to four days after he said he was getting rid of her, she was gone. I didn't know where, but I was glad he hadn't asked me to put her down, as some people would have done. Of course, for all I knew, he may have sent her to the dog food people, but I hoped not.

A few days later, Jim-2 called. He rarely called; his mare had been bred in late March and was safely in foal, so I hadn't expected to hear from him until at least the first of the year.

"Doc, I got a new mare and I wanna breed her," he said.

My first thought was that he couldn't afford another mare. He always paid, but he was very slow about it because he just didn't have the money. But how and what he spent were not my decisions. "It's nearly July, Jim," I told him. "Why don't you wait 'til next year?"

But he insisted he wanted to breed her, so I went out to the few acres he leased. He led out a very large, very coarse plain bay mare that looked remarkably familiar, but I couldn't quite place her. I checked and cultured her

When I finished, I began writing up the ticket. "What's her name, Jim?" I asked.

"I don't remember," he replied, "I just got her a couple days ago. I'll let you know next time."

"Next time" was two days later. The culture was clean, so we checked her for a breeding date. As I was palpating her, I commented, "This mare sure looks familiar."

"She's just a plain bay mare, Doc. A lot of 'em look a lot alike."

As I was writing up the ticket, I asked again, "What's her name?"

"Peon's Poem," he said.

Oh, no, I thought. Jim-1 could afford big vet bills; Jim-2 couldn't. I didn't have the heart to tell him about her.

"How'd you get her?" I asked weakly. He told me his friend Jim-1 gave her to him. Some friend, I thought.

Peon's Poem got in foal from that breeding, had a normal pregnancy, and produced a beautiful colt the next June. Jim-2 decided to sell the colt as a yearling. He had received a complimentary (i.e., free) service to a mediocre stallion; nonetheless, the colt, because of his looks and the performance of Peon's Poem's other foal, sold for $18,000.

Peon's Poem was never dirty again. She died at fourteen from a serious colic, but gave Jim-2 three foals in five years, not great production but certainly better than she had given Jim-1. He was absolutely delighted with her.

Jim-1 was angry and moved Flo and Buttered Toast, and another mare he had replaced Peon's Poem with, to another farm so I couldn't work on them. It got back to me that he had told some people that I had worked this out with Jim-2 and that's why I wouldn't let Peon's Poem get in foal for him.

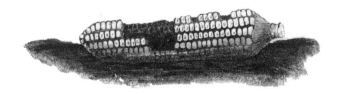

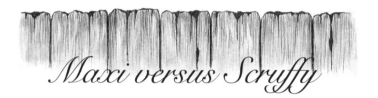

Maxi versus Scruffy

PEOPLE HAVE ASKED ME what my favorite animal is. They mean species, not individual specimen. It's a tough question.

We can eliminate cows from consideration, but that doesn't really narrow the field much because there are still a jillion species remaining. I love horses, but not many horses reciprocate. Pigs are neat and they do reciprocate—or some do—but I've never had a pet pig. Even though I like them, they're just a little bit overwhelming on a one-on-one basis.

Goats are too capricious (I like that word), sheep are too stupid; birds and fish are too impersonal (although ducks are wonderful); wild animals aren't even considered because they should stay in the wild. That pretty much narrows it down to cats and dogs, which I guess, is why darn near all my classmates are small-animal vets.

I think cats inspire more emotion than any other species. No—I know it. There are dog lovers and horse lovers, and probably somewhere in a padded cell, a cow lover, but rarely are they fanatical. There are also haters of these species, but usually their hatred simply causes them to avoid those animals they hate.

But cats! Cat lovers amass cats the way little boys amass baseball cards (but baseball cards don't need a litter box). I've known "cat people" who owned literally dozens of their chosen passion.

Cat haters don't just simply avoid cats—they often go out of their way to hurt or kill them. And usually there's no reason for their hatred; they hate them simply because they're cats. (I have never understood hatred in general and, more specifically, hating something—or someone—just because of what he/she/it/they is/are.)

Through the centuries, societies and civilizations have revered, even idolized, cats; others have feared and shunned and persecuted them. Other domestic animals have rarely received these "honors."

Several years ago I wrote a magazine article that was particularly good to me: I sold it, in slightly modified form, three times. It was on the care of barn cats.

The first sale was to a Canadian magazine geared to weekend or gentlemen farmers. The editor forwarded a couple of letters it inspired. One was from a woman whose praise was unbounded. She wanted to use my name in a campaign to promote proper care of Canadian barn cats. I wrote back and thanked her for her interest but declined, although I found it interesting to picture this lady trudging through northern Manitoba, possibly in January, telling farmers and ranchers, "Dr. Kendall says to take better care of your barn cats!"

The second sale was to a magazine aimed at southern farm families. This time, I received a letter (again forwarded to me by the editor) from a woman in Tennessee. She was irate that I would suggest that cats should be placed in such a "dangerous" environment as a barn. "They should be kept in the house," she wrote. "There are large farm animals and machinery that could hurt them," she pointed out. "And what about dogs?" she asked.

I wrote to her and told her that I thought it was unfair to keep a cat, or any animal, always in the house. "And besides," I wrote, "dogs don't make good mousers."

Well, her second letter was even more irate. I must be a terrible vet, she informed me, and she felt sorry for my clients. (So do I, sometimes.) The crack about dogs really upset her. "You know very well what I mean!" she wrote.

The third sale was to a horse industry publication. A letter from a man in Oregon was forwarded to me. It began, "I don't hate cats, but I see no reason for their existence." It turned out he is a militant bird-watcher. Later on in his letter, he explained how he traps feral cats and shoots them. He was kind enough to understand that perhaps not all people would want to shoot these cats, so he thoughtfully told, in detail, how to poison them. I didn't respond to this guy. I didn't want someone who kills things he doesn't hate to know my address.

I'm very fond of cats. Some I have loved. Annie was wonderful. Calico, from my childhood, was possibly the world's most loved cat. Ray, an old Manx I've never written about, was a marvelous cat. But enough cats have taken my hospitality and my food and given nothing in return, so cats, even though I can't imagine being without at least one, are not my favorites.

That leaves dogs. I think all dogs, given the chance and treated properly, would love a master. All are not given that chance, unfortunately, and too many just aren't treated properly.

And all dogs aren't for all people, which is one of the reasons there are so many breeds. Another reason, of course, is function—what they were originally bred to do. A Pomeranian could not take the role of a Rhodesian Ridgeback, for instance, whose job it is to hunt lions.

Over the years, I've owned several breeds of various sizes, from a 140-pound Saint Bernard down to an 8-pound Bichon Frise, and each one, with the significant exception of Soldier, the Doberman, has been a wonderful, loving, and protecting (yes, even Peep, the Bichon, would attempt to protect us from evil-doers such as the UPS man, the meter readers, etc.) pet.

All our dogs have not been purebreds. Also in the mix have been a number of mutts, ranging from a 70-pound probably part-Shepherd named Ranger down to a 20-pound you-name-it named Beauregard, who is probably one of my three all-time favorites (the other two being Squirrel and Orf, also mutts on the small side).

Even though I have loved our big dogs, they have actually been my wife's choices. I have always preferred small (but not tiny) dogs. I've had a few Fox Terriers over the past eons, and that is (or maybe was) my favorite breed. I like their intelligence and personality in addition to their size.

A few years ago, we found ourselves without a small dog. Beauregard had been accidentally killed, and we were left with Cleo, a Ridgeback, and Bastille, a Labrador Retriever. I hate to admit it, but I grieved for months over Beau's death and I think I went into a depression. I still become very sad when I think of the little guy; his passing hit me harder than that of any other.

I guess it showed because my wife suggested frequently that I get another small dog, but I was steadfast in my refusal. I guess I figured I couldn't stay morose and depressed at a proper level of misery if I had reason not to.

After a couple of years of this and in spite of my objections, the kids (spurred, no doubt, and probably financed by my wife) surprised me one Christmas with a scroungy little rat of a puppy, "rat" being the operative word. It was an almost six-week-old rat terrier.

She was pot-bellied from parasites and lethargic and very lucky because I don't think she would have lived much longer if the kids hadn't bought her and removed her from her previous environment. Worming did wonders for her, and with two or three days of TLC she was a different puppy. I named her Mini because of her size. When her health and condition improved, so did her personality and activity.

She had—and still has—only two modes of action: coma and frenzy. There is no, or very little, transitional phase. When she's asleep, she appears to be dead, and when she's awake, she's a blur.

And she's very intelligent. I have always believed terriers were smart dogs, in spite of their seeming scatter-brained personalities, and Mini has done nothing but reinforce that belief.

At the risk of being accused of not staying on a subject, I will now skip to another for a moment. The old man who lives in the small house on the property that adjoins ours owned a large, old, orange tomcat named Bud. Bud was an excellent cat; he came to visit us frequently, sometimes daily, and would even come in the house if he found an open door. He spent many nights in our garage, accidentally closed in, but he never minded. We'd find him in the mornings, asleep on or in one of the cars.

The cats pretty much ignored Bud and the dogs didn't seem to mind him or he them. He was more or less a part of the landscape as far as all the animals were concerned.

I will now appear to change subjects again. Mini needed to be watched when she went outside in her younger days. Early on, a hungry red-tailed hawk, finding slim pickings in the cold days of winter, had made a swoop at her, but luckily our daughter stepped outside at that moment and the hawk altered its course. Mini had seen it coming and was justifiably frightened. She weighed 3 pounds max and was just the right size for a decent meal.

From that point, one of us would accompany her when she needed to go out. I was the one with her when she first discovered Bud. She knew the house cats and had pretty much accepted them, but this was something new. She took off after the old cat, barking fiercely. Or at least, as fiercely as a 3-pound puppy can bark. Bud turned and ran.

I don't profess to know what goes on in animals' minds, so all I can do is anthropomorphize. Bud was a *big* cat, probably 15 to 16 pounds, and I imagine that occurred to him. Hey, he must have thought, I'm a *big* cat! That thing chasing me is hardly bite-sized.

So Bud stopped. When he stopped, Mini stopped. Then Bud turned and jumped at Mini and she took off as fast as she could. Old Bud could have caught her but he didn't. That became a game between the two: Mini would chase Bud, then Bud would chase her. It happened four or five times a week, whenever they would encounter each other outside.

Mini grew to an eventual 12 pounds and safe from hawks, and I kept telling the family I was going to breed her. My wife couldn't understand why I would want to reproduce something so useless. (I've felt that way about many people I've known when I heard of the births of their heirs.) Rat terriers, however, are not the most common breed, and I never found a male and immaculate conception, even in a Christmas gift, just doesn't occur, so Mini turned two and still retained her maidenhood.

The local cat population, unfortunately, experienced some drastic and tragic alterations as Mini was growing. We found Fang lying dead in the second horse, *né* tobacco, barn. He had no marks on him; we think he must have fallen from a rafter. If you recall, Fang fell easily and often.

Gary, who, to the best of our knowledge, had never gone in the road, did so one day. It may not have been the first time, but it was the last. (I really miss her.) Tumbleweed, heretofore unmentioned, may have met his demise in the same manner, but we don't know. He just disappeared.

A new cat showed up one day, from where we have no idea. Like Bud and the aforementioned Ralphie, he was—is—an orange tom of unbelievable pacifity. "Laid back" is a fitting description. We named him Scruffy because of his appearance, and nothing fazed him for the first year of his presence in our household.

And then the road claimed Bud. My wife saw it happen, but I was the one who had to tell Mr. Winkle, his owner. Except for occasional visits from his daughter and her children, Mr. Winkle's only companion had been old Bud. I thought the old gentleman was going to faint when I told him. I asked if he wanted another cat—I could easily get a kitten for him, and his daughter tried to convince him to take one—but he always just said, "No," and wouldn't discuss it.

Mini's second birthday came, and still no boyfriend for her was in sight. Christmas was on the horizon and I overheard the kids—"kids" is no longer applicable, they're adults—talking. They were going to give me a male rat terrier puppy.

Okay, so I knew what I was getting for Christmas, but I'd still act surprised. I began thinking of names. Mini is small, so would a male be, I reasoned. I'd call him Micro.

Christmas came and with it the introduction of this male Rat Terrier puppy. I acted surprised, but it wasn't an act as it turned out. I was expecting something along the lines of Mini—small and delicate with a racehorse build—but instead I was presented with a ten-week-old behemoth that was already larger than Mini was at two years. I quickly changed his name to Maxi. (My daughter says the two—Mini and Maxi—sound like feminine hygiene products.)

And Maxi grew and grew. If Mini is a racehorse—lean, sleek, svelte: a Thoroughbred—then Maxi is a draft horse—stocky, blocky, huge, cumbersome: a Clydesdale. (For those readers not fully conversant with horse breeds, picture instead a ballerina and a Sumo wrestler.)

Poor Maxi had apparently only been handled when being wormed or vaccinated because he was afraid of everything, especially people, but the ever-important TLC brought him around in a couple of weeks. And with that coming-around came a level of aggression we hadn't expected: He wasn't a "Rat" Terrier, he was a "cat" terrier. He didn't hurt them, but he loved to jump on them and act as if he would tear them apart. Old Nixon, not previously mentioned but remarkable only for his uncanny ability to barf nearly every day, simply retreated to a safe level—a countertop or chair—but laid-back Scruffy just held his ground and meowed pitifully, which he would do whenever he saw Maxi approaching—*before* actual contact was made—so we knew he wasn't hurting him. And he never had any marks on him after a Maxi "attack."

But it was aggravating him. After a few weeks of this, he began staying away for a day, then two. We didn't know where he went and we worried about him, but he'd always return eventually, only to be mauled again by Maxi.

One day, Roberta, Mr. Winkle's daughter, stopped by. "I just wanted to tell you not to worry about your cat," she said.

I wasn't sure what she meant, so I said as much.

"The orange one," she explained. "He spends three or four days a week with Daddy. He just walked in one day when we were visiting and the kids left the door open. Daddy says he's not his cat so he's not going to buy any cat food but he feeds him tuna instead."

And that's the way it's remained: Scruffy spends about half his time with Mr. Winkle. He comes home—or I should say, to us—for a little dry cat food and his obligatory mauling by Maxi, but then goes over for his tuna and the peace and serenity of watching TV with Mr. Winkle.

When Mini has puppies, that will probably drive him to Mr. Winkle full time. He couldn't have a better home. But maybe I'll give Mr. Winkle a rat terrier puppy. Maybe that will get Scruffy to come back.

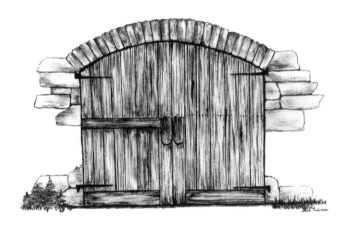

$\mathcal{G}$LOSSARY

Anabolic Describes a process in animals by which food is converted to tissue. Also an agent that builds the body.

Barren Describes a mare that was bred but did not conceive.

Bay A horse color, light to dark brown with black mane, tail, and lower legs.

Black type Boldfaced print; used on a catalog page to indicate a stakes performer.

Blinkers Cups or flaps attached to the bridle that prevent a horse from using his peripheral vision so he won't be distracted.

Book (v.) To arrange for the mating of a mare to a stallion.

Breaking The initial training given a young horse so it may be ridden.

Breeding shed A building, often attached to a barn, used solely for the mating of mares to stallions.

Broodmare A female horse used for foal production.

Cannon The bone between the knee (front) or hock (rear) and the ankle of a horse.

Chestnut   A horse color, yellowish to reddish to brown with mane, tail, and lower legs of the same color.

Claimer/claiming race   A horse for sale in a claiming race, which is a cheap class of race. A horse entered in a claiming race may be "claimed" by another owner for the claiming price.

Coggins test   A blood test to determine if a horse is positive for equine infectious anemia, a disease spread by biting insects.

Colic   Signs of abdominal distress; not a specific disease.

Colostrum   "First milk"; necessary for the newborn because it contains important antibodies.

Coronet   The area where the hoof meets the ankle.

Cover   (*v.*) To breed a mare.

Cradle   A method to move a horse that doesn't want to move; two people lock arms across the horse's rear and pull him forward.

Culture   A test to see if there are bacteria present.

Diuretic   A drug that causes an increase in urination.

Dystocia   Difficult parturition.

Ear   (*v.*) To grab a horse's ear and squeeze or twist it; a way to control a fractious animal.

Estrous cycle   The time from one ovulation to the next; typically about three weeks in mares.

Euthanasia   Humane destruction.

Farrier   A blacksmith.

Farrow   (*n.*) A baby pig; (*v.*) to have a litter of pigs.

Foal heat   The first heat period a mare has after foaling; usually at eight to twelve days later.

Follicle   A balloonlike structure that arises on an ovary; it contains the egg.

Furlong   One-eighth of a mile; used to measure horse races.

Gelding   A male horse that has been castrated.

Gravel   The term for an infection that enters a horse's foot at the sole and migrates upward until it erupts at the coronet.

Growth medium   A mixture of nutrients conducive to bacterial growth.

Hot walker   A person who walks a horse that needs to be cooled out after having been raced or trained.

In foal   Pregnant; a pregnant mare is said to be "in foal."

In heat (in season)   Receptive to the male for breeding.

Jockey Club, The   The governing body, rules-making organ, and registration center of the Thoroughbred horse industry.

Jump   The mounting of a mare by a teaser to see if she will hold still to be bred.

Lay-up   (*n.*) A horse brought from the racetrack to the farm for a period of time to recover from illness or injury.

Let-down   (*n.*) The transition period for horses between the rigors of training and the relative ease of farm life.

Lights   Artificially lengthening the amount of daylight by putting mares in lighted stalls; it causes the mares to begin cycling earlier.

Lube   A viscous, water-soluble material used primarily to make rectal palpation safer and easier.

Maiden   A horse (of either sex) that has not won a race; also a mare that has never been bred.

Mastitis   Inflammation of the udder.

On the board   Finishing first, second, third, or fourth in a horse race; the first four finishers are listed on the tote board.

Ovulation   The release of the egg from the follicle.

Palp/palpate   To reach in rectally and feel the internal organs, specifically the ovaries and uterus, in a reproductive exam.

Parasite ova   Worm eggs.

Parturition   Giving birth.

Peristalsis   The normal, involuntary movement of the gastrointestinal tract.

Peritoneal cavity   The potential space between the layers of the peritoneum, the lining of the abdominal cavity.

Peritonitis   Inflammation or infection of the peritoneum.

Progesterone   A hormone necessary for the maintenance of pregnancy.

Pubis   One of the pelvic bones.

Quarter crack   A crack in the hoof wall on the side of the foot, which is termed the "quarter."

Registration certificate   Proof that a Thoroughbred has been recorded with the Jockey Club; necessary for racing or breeding.

Ridgling   A horse with one or both testicles retained within the body cavity.

RNA   Ribonucleic acid, which is important in genetic transmission; in horse sales summaries, it means "Reserve Not Attained."

Savage   (*v.*) The action of a horse that bites, or attempts to bite, another horse or person.

Shank/lead shank   A rope or strap used to lead a horse.

Show   (*v.*) To respond positively to a teaser; to run third in a race.

Slip   To abort.

Spay   To remove the reproductive organs of a female.

Speculum (*n.*)/ spec. (*v.*) A tube used to visualize the vagina and cervix; to examine by using a speculum.

Stakes race   The highest class of horse race; a stakes race has a purse value that is made up of a given amount plus the entry fees paid by owners to enter their horses.

Stall mucker   A person whose job it is to clean stalls.

Stopping a mare   Getting a mare in foal.

Suture   To repair a laceration or, in mares, to partially close the vulva to prevent external contamination of the vagina, cervix, and uterus.

Tail/tail up   To forcibly elevate the tail over an animal's back by grasping it very close to the body and pushing upward; prevents kicking in most cases.

Tear   A vulvar laceration incurred during foaling.

Tease   (*v.*) To see if a mare is in season by exposing her to a teaser.

Teaser   A male horse used to see if mares are in season.

Teratogenicity   The ability of a drug to cause fetal malformations.

Third eyelid   The nictitating membrane; a membrane in the inner corner of horses' eyes.

Thoroughbred-cross   A horse with one Thoroughbred parent and one non-Thoroughbred parent.

Transport medium   A mixture of nutrients that sustain bacterial life until a culture swab can be taken to a laboratory.

Weanling   A young horse from the time it is taken off its dam through December 31 of the year of birth.

Withers   The highest part of a horse's back, just behind the neck.

Worm/deworm   (*v.*) To give a medication that kills internal parasites.

Yearling   A one-year-old horse. Any horse between January 1 and December 31 of the year *after* it is born.